100 **great** *natural* **remedies**

penelope ody

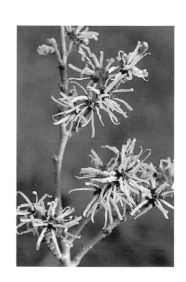

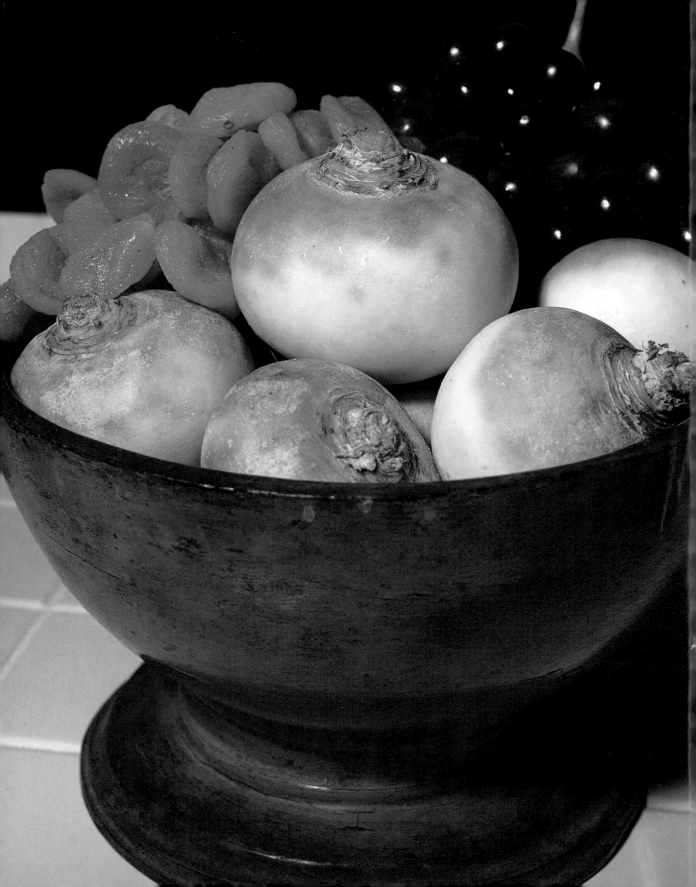

100 **great**

natural

remedies

Using Healing Plants at Home

Penelope Ody

Kyle Cathie Limited

For John Clive as always

First published in Great Britain in 1997 by
Kyle Cathie Limited,
20 Vauxhall Bridge Road
London SW1V 2SA

ISBN 1 85626 257 X

Original photography by Laura Hodgson
Designed by Geoff Hayes
Edited by Caroline Taggart
See also photographic acknowledgements on page 192

Penelope Ody is hereby identified as the author of this work in accordance with Section 77 of the Copyright, Designs and Patents Act 1988.

A Cataloguing in Publication record for this title is available from the British Library.

Printed in Singapore by Tien Wah Press

Half-title page: Witch hazel Hamamelis virginiana

contents

All nature is like one single apothecary's shop, covered only with the roof of heaven; and only One Being works the pestle as far as the world extends. But man has such a shop only in part, not wholly; he possesses something, not everything. For nature's apothecary's shop is greater than man's.

Paracelsus (1493-1541)

Acknowledgements

Thanks are especially due to Caroline Taggart for her patient and unflappable editing and imaginative picture sourcing; to Deni Bown, whose meticulous taxonomy has provided herbalists with a definitive guide to botanical names; to numerous herbal colleagues over many years whose chance remarks and favourite remedies have added to my own stockpile of knowledge; and to my grandmother, Mary Hannah Tweddell (1879-1963), whose homespun remedies based on the ingredients of her kitchen cupboard first made me aware of what useful healing tools we all have readily to hand.

Important note

The information and advice contained in this book are intended as a general guide to using plants and are not specific to individuals or their particular circumstances. Many plant substances, whether sold as foods or as medicines and used externally or internally, can cause an allergic reaction in some people. Neither the author nor the publishers can be held responsible for claims arising from the inappropriate use of any remedy or healing regime. Do not attempt self-diagnosis or self-treatment for serious or long-term conditions before consulting a medical professional or qualified practitioner. Do not undertake any self-treatment while taking other prescribed drugs or receiving therapy without first seeking professional guidance. Always seek medical advice if any symptoms persist.

introduction: **using** nature's **medicines**

Until the arrival of low-cost, state-sponsored health care and potent, readily-available pharmaceutical drugs, the only medicines available to most people were the ones that could be found in the local wood, meadow or physic garden. Plant medicines have been in regular, well-documented use for at least 5,000 years and probably much longer: there is evidence that many mammals will seek out and eat particular plants when they feel ill and who is to know whether or not our cave-dwelling ancestors did exactly the same? Indeed, traces of medicinal herbs like yarrow and marshmallow have been found in Neanderthal graves of 65,000 years ago, suggesting at least some contemporary significance for these plants.

Our Western tradition of herbal medicine is largely derived from Greek and Roman practice, with many herbs used today much as they were by Dioscorides – a surgeon with Nero's army who wrote one of our earliest surviving herbals in the first century AD. Greek medicine, as originally described by Hippocrates, the "father of modern medicine" (c. 460–c. 370 BC), was based on the belief that all matter is made up of four elements: earth, air, fire and water. These elements had their own characteristics and qualities: "earth", for example, was regarded as heavy, stable and firm, while "fire" travels upwards, intermingles and permeates all things. The Greeks applied the concept of elements to

the four bodily fluids or "humours" which early physicians had identified. These were "blood", associated with air; "phlegm", linked with water; "yellow bile" or the "choleric humour" – fire; and "black bile", corresponding to earth. Like the elements, these humours had to be kept in balance and excess was believed to lead to ill health. Those suffering from a surfeit of black bile (described as "melancholic") would have been given strong purgatives as the resulting diarrhoea was visible evidence of removal of excess of this particular humour from the system. Those with too much blood (sanguine) were good humoured but prone to over-indulgence – hence the habit of "bleeding" patients.

The humoral model was codified by Galen (AD 131–199), so is often termed "Galenical medicine". With the fall of the Roman Empire in the fifth century, this Greek tradition was kept alive by the Arabs and was further refined and developed by such notable physicians as Avicenna al-Hussain (Abdullah Ibn Sina, died 1037). Today, it survives in the Tibb or Unani medical tradition, which is practised throughout the Islamic world.

Avicenna's work was highly regarded by later European herbalists and was widely quoted by herbal writers until well into the 18th century, when Galenical theories began to be replaced by a more modern approach to medicine.

When it came to identifying plant properties, these early herbalists had largely to depend on trial and error, but to support the guesswork they used a theory known as the "Doctrine of Signatures". This maintained that the appearance of plants provided clues to their properties. Yellow-flowered plants such as dandelion were believed to be good for treating jaundice, for example, while the nodular roots of lesser celandine (*Ranunculus ficaria*) were said to resemble piles, giving the plant its country name of pilewort. Both pilewort and dandelion live up to their signatures and are used, respectively, for treating piles and liver disorders today.

While many associated the "doctrine" with the noted German herbalist Paracelsus (1493–1541), similar theories are found in many cultures. The Chinese, for example, recommend cinnamon twigs to warm the hands and toes, while the tree trunk's bark is more suitable for warming the body.

In Galenical theory, elements and humours were also defined in terms of cold or hot, dry or damp: earth and black bile, for example, were both cold and dry, while blood was – understandably – hot and moist. Herbs were similarly classified and over the centuries the descriptions became ever more sophisticated with several "degrees" of hotness, dampness and so on.

The great Elizabethan herbalist John Gerard, writing in 1597, tells us that horseradish is "hot and dry in the third degree". It would therefore have been used to combat severe problems of cold and damp – excess phlegm – by restoring the balance. In contrast chickweed is "cold and moist and of a waterish substance", so would be helpful with problems of heat and dryness, such as the dry, scaling, irritant eczema for which it is still recommended today.

Just as herbs were characterised on this elemental basis, so too were foods; housewives would take care to balance their meals in terms of temperature and moisture content. The Italian Giacomo Castelvetro, writing in 1614, urges the use of pepper as a seasoning for numerous cold and damp vegetables – such as beans – which would otherwise cause wind and stomach upsets, and recommends a walnut sauce (reasonably hot and dry) for pork "as an antidote to its harmful qualities". Certain foods – such as cucumber and strawberries – were known to increase cold and damp humours, so would be avoided in winter when the prevailing climate was already doing just that.

With the coming of the Industrial Revolution and the population drift from countryside to towns and cities, this sort of knowledge was gradually lost. By the 1850s, the emphasis was firmly on patent remedies, and a new generation of urban poor had little help when it came to illness.

The typhoid and cholera epidemics associated with Victorian slums did, however, help encourage a herbal revival with an influx of American-trained "herb and root" doctors, who brought new plants and healing techniques from the New World. Albert Coffin and Wooster Beech arrived from the United States with their messages of "Physiomedicalism" and "Eclecticism" – movements founded in 18th-century New England and derived, in part, from the Galenical model combined with Native American traditions of sweat houses and heating remedies. Samuel Thomson, founder of the Physiomedical movement, believed that all disease was caused by cold and he used sweat treatments combined with emetics and purgatives to clear the system of cold and damp phlegm.

The message proved extremely popular in the newly industrialised towns of Northern England, where Eclectic herbalists thrived until well into the 1930s. Many traditional over-the-counter products are still based on these North American theories, with extensive use of herbs such as chili to warm the system. Many American herbs, such as golden seal, were introduced to the British herbal *materia medica* at this time, and while these plants remain popular in the UK, there is often little tradition of using them in other parts of Europe where Physiomedicalism never penetrated.

The Eclectic influence encouraged renewed interest in herbal medicine – although in remedies purchased from specialist herb shops in urban areas rather than in home-grown products or attempts at harvesting from the wild, so the old traditions continued to decline.

Today, mainstream herbal medicine has embraced other new and fashionable influences as Ayurvedic and traditional Chinese products enter the marketplace. A few years ago it was virtually impossible to buy Chinese herbs in Europe. The intrepid could venture into Soho's Chinatown and similar centres and, if the language problems were not insurmountable, emerge with a bag of miscellaneous brown things which may or may not have been what they wanted. Today, Chinese herbs are being tested in state hospitals and Chinese "doctors" thrive in numerous high-street shops and clinics.

Traditional Chinese medicine is, like Galenical theory, based on a model that links elements with bodily functions. In this case there are five elements (earth, wood, fire, water and metal) related to the five main organs of the body (spleen, liver, heart, kidney, and lungs), five emotions, fluids, tastes (sweet, sour, bitter, salty and pungent) and so on. Herbs are defined by taste and temperature, which links them to associated body organs and function. Sweet herbs, for example, are nutritious and tonifying for the stomach; salty herbs are associated with fluid balance and kidney function.

As well as the five-element model, the Chinese also believe in the duality of vital energy or *Qi* (sometimes spelt *ch'i*), which has both *yang* and *yin* aspects. *Yang* is associated with the male, light and heat, whereas *yin* is seen as female, dark and cold. Herbs are similarly divided: Korean ginseng, for example, is a *yang* tonic; American ginseng is considered as benefiting *yin* energy.

A number of Chinese herbs are now being included in mainstream herbal products. Ginseng has been available for years, but a newcomer is *Dang Gui* (Chinese angelica), which is defined in Chinese theory as a blood tonic, and there is also considerable interest in the medicinal fungi used in China.

The oriental fashion is also influencing herbal product suppliers and a number of Chinese-style over-the-counter remedies are now appearing which contain plants that would have been quite unfamiliar to our grandmothers. We can, however, easily benefit from this Eastern knowledge when it is combined with the trend for grocery exotica. The shiitake mushroom (see page 101) – now to be found on supermarket shelves up and down the country – is an extremely potent tonic and immune-stimulating herb with an impressive array of medical properties which make this comparatively unfamiliar vegetable well worth adding to the household medicine chest.

Indian Ayurvedic theory is a combination of very ancient health and philosophical traditions – dating back to around 5,000 BC – overlaid by later Islamic influence and Unani (Greek) medicine. Like Galenical medicine,

Ayurveda is based on a model of bodily humours (*doshas*) and a need to maintain the inner life force (*prana*) which is believed to give rise to the fire of digestion and mental energy. *Prana* is linked to breath or oxygen which feeds the fire and, if the fire is weak, then the body is weak.

Around 800 herbs are used in the "great tradition" of Ayurvedic medicine, although there is also a strong regional folk tradition covering around 2,500 medicinal herbs which are used in what is known as the "lesser medicine". Each household has its own *maharastra* or "grandmother's purse", filled with healing herbs for the household, and the traditions of how to use these have been passed continuously from mother to daughter for generations in the manner of native healers everywhere.

Ayurvedic medicine is less well known in Europe than Chinese traditional medicine, but is growing in popularity: herbs worth investigating include *gotu kola* (*Centella asiatica*), known in India as *brahmi*, which is one of Ayurveda's most important tonic herbs, long used as a rejuvenating remedy to counter the problems of old age and improve failing memory. Basil (*Ocimum basilicum*), used in the West mainly to season tomato and pasta dishes, is another of the great Ayurvedic tonics, considered as giving divine protection, spiritually healing and strengthening for the immune system and "vital force".

Choosing natural remedies

For many people in the West the label "herb" conjures up a fairly stereotyped image of something aromatic and green, probably used for flavouring and sometimes displaying medicinal properties. The *Shorter Oxford English Dictionary* confirms the imagery: "…plants of which the leaves, or stem and leaves, are used for food or medicine, or for their scent and flavour".

We can, however, put a great many more items into the "natural remedies" category than a few archetypal "herbs". Chinese medicine, for example, is notorious for its use of animal parts and the macabre practices of suppliers trying to obtain them, while Ayurvedic cures contain a wide assortment of minerals and metals – not all of them ones that would be considered perfectly safe or savoury by Westerners.

Staying with plants, we can also add plenty of other items to the dictionary definition. There are the fruits – such as hawthorn berries, used in medicine, and juniper berries, which good cooks regularly add to game dishes and terrines – and plenty of roots like ginseng and horseradish which most people would accept as "herbs". Fungi, too, may be less often used medicinally in the West than in China, but the flavoursome virtues of truffles or the therapeutic properties of shiitake cannot be denied. And then there are flowers: calendula cream made from marigold petals is a popular antiseptic, while chamomile flower tea is a favourite relaxing drink with many people.

Separating "food" from "plant medicine" is no easy task either: the garlic sold on the greengrocer's counter is technically "food", but the same cloves could just as easily be prescribed as a heart tonic or to combat candidiasis. Today's appreciation of plant properties has seen a spate of recommendations and media headlines urging us to eat broccoli or carrots to help protect against cancer, to drink wine to combat heart disease or to fight depression with St John's wort. Are we talking here of "foods" or "medicines"?

Medicinal herbs can be, and often are, used as foods or culinary flavourings, and what nicer way to take your daily dose than in a warming cup of tea or spicing the evening's meal? Equally, one must remember that foods often have a potent therapeutic effect and that some – in high doses – can be extremely toxic. It is unlikely that if the potato were discovered today it would be passed as fit for human consumption because of the poisonous alkaloids it contains.

In the past knowledge of the healing properties and use of plants was something handed down between generations: the family "receipt" book with its mixture of supper dishes, jams and cough mixtures was commonplace and brewing up a healing gruel to combat colds and chills was as much a part of everyday life as baking a cake. The seasonal use of particular plants was common knowledge, as was the intrinsic character of the food and flavourings – be they hot, damp, dry or cooling – and the likely effect it could have on healthy natural balance.

Today, central heating, air conditioning and air-freighted exotic foods tend to make our living conditions and diet much the same throughout the year and we have forgotten not only the healing skills of our great-grandmothers, but nature's own rhythms as well. Most people would regard gathering wild plants and eating them as a certain way of contracting food poisoning: we have lost both the confidence to use nature's remedies and the intuitive skill to know when we need them.

Herbal remedies in the home

We live in an age of "magic bullets" where medicine is something powerful, shrink-wrapped and "guaranteed" to clear symptoms in hours rather than days; to "bring instant relief" or make us "feel better – faster", as the advertisements usually proclaim. The idea that well-being requires personal effort and involvement is as alien to many people as the concept of using beans, rather than highly processed granules, to make coffee.

We also live in an age when many of us have too many things to do and too little time in which to do them; where the key word in food shopping is "convenience" and the recipe writers tell us that life is too short to stuff a mushroom.

In such a world it is hardly surprising that gathering herbs, drying them slowly and carefully at home, and then taking the time and trouble to blend them to make healing teas, or spend hours over a hot stove stirring creams and ointments, seems to belong to another age. Yet it is just this sort of involvement that is needed if we are really to heal ourselves.

Rather than expect the health-care professional – be that an orthodox general practitioner or a herbal specialist – to prescribe a wonder cure, we need to take responsibility for our own well being. Taking the time to brew skullcap and lemon balm tea at the end of a busy day, and then do nothing but sip it for 10 minutes, is just as valuable for the over-stressed sufferer as the herbs' sedative properties. Active involvement in our own cure is essential. As a practitioner, I all too often encounter patients who are happy to try herbal medicine, but are unwilling to spend time taking even a little exercise – those who burn the candle at both ends and then expect a herbal tonic to restore the imbalances in their bodily system that they have themselves created.

Taking responsibility for your health means listening to your body: learning to identify the early signs of illness – the sore throat that will turn into laryngitis, for example, or the minor twinge that could become a frozen shoulder – and taking action at that stage, rather than waiting until professional help is the only solution. Obviously there are times when urgent medical attention is essential, but for the sort of commonplace, self-limiting ailments that send some people to their local chemist for over-the-counter cures and others to their GP's surgery for yet another course of antibiotics ·or tranquillisers, natural home remedies can provide the ideal alternative.

This book cannot pretend to be comprehensive – there are many thousands of plants with therapeutic properties and several hundred of these could be used as household remedies. Instead it focuses on over 100 readily available plant products – be they found on greengrocer's counter, growing wild in the countryside or neatly labelled as herbal medicines in the health-food shop. But by looking at a cross-section of the herbs, foods and wild flowers that can be used in making simple home remedies, the book might just encourage a little more willingness to take responsibility for our own health and confidence to use some of these readily available medicines.

Cautions

People are fond of saying that "herbal medicine is safer". Certainly herbs can have fewer side effects than some orthodox drugs but, as Paracelsus always reminded us, everything is toxic to a greater or lesser degree. Just because herbs are "natural plants" rather than laboratory-concocted chemicals does not mean that they are totally harmless. Healing plants are powerful and need to be treated with respect.

When gathering plants from the wild, always check identification very carefully and when planning to grow at home don't assume that a plant has been correctly labelled by the nursery or seedsman. Use a good wildflower key or illustrated herbal to confirm the identity of your plants. I once planted a packet of catmint seeds (*Nepeta cataria*) which when fully grown proved to be marsh woundwort.

When using ready-made products always follow recommended dosages and never exceed the general guidelines given in Part 1. Always seek professional help for any persistent symptoms or if there is a sudden change in condition as well as for acute pain or prolonged high temperatures.

A few herbs can conflict with orthodox medication – such as feverfew with blood-thinning drugs – so seek professional advice if you are on long-term medication and would like to use home-made remedies.

Similarly the list of herbs to avoid in pregnancy can appear excessively long but in most cases concern is over high, therapeutic doses. A few of the herbs listed have been reported to cause foetal abnormalities, but most act as uterine stimulants so can increase the risk of miscarriage. As a general rule avoid taking any medication (herbal or otherwise) during the first three months of pregnancy unless recommended to do so by your health-care professional.

Plants to avoid totally in pregnancy are: arbor vitae (*Thuja occidentalis*), barberry (*Berberis vulgaris*), basil oil (*Ocimum basilicum*), black cohosh (*Cimicifuga racemosus*), blue cohosh (*Caulophyllum thalictroides*), chamomile oil, Dang Gui (*Angelica polymorpha* var. *sinensis*), feverfew, golden seal, greater celandine, juniper, lady's mantle (*Alchemilla vulgaris*), mistletoe (*Viscum album*), motherwort (*Leonurus cardiaca*), mugwort (*Artemisia vulgaris*), myrrh (*Commiphora molmol*), pennyroyal (*Mentha pulegium*), pokeroot (*Phytolacca decandra*), rue (*Ruta graveolens*), shepherd's purse, southernwood (*Artemisia abrotanum*), tansy (*Tanacetum vulgare*) and wormwood (*Artemisia absinthium*).

Avoid regular large or therapeutic doses of the following: angelica (*Angelica archangelica*), bitter orange, chili, celery seed, cinnamon, cowslip (*Primula veris*), elder bark, fennel, fenugreek (*Trigonella foenum-graecum*), Korean ginseng, lavender, marjoram (*Origanum vulgare*), nutmeg, parsley, rhubarb root (*Rheum palmatum*), senna (*Senna alexandrina*), sage, thyme, vervain, wild yam (*Dioscorea villosa*), wood betony and yarrow. (Botanical names are given only for those herbs not included in Part 2 of this book.)

part 1: making and buying natural remedies

Herbal medicine has always been a "medicine of the people" – simple, easily found plant or vegetable remedies that could be brewed at home to treat a wide variety of ailments. For all too many of us today those remedies are no longer quite so easily found. Urban lifestyles make gathering wild plants a rare experience, while the pressures of modern life mean that few of us have spare time to make creams and tinctures for home use.

Rediscovering some of the old household healing arts is not difficult. Simple remedies can be made quickly in the kitchen and even if access to the countryside is limited we can still grow healing plants in the garden or buy dried supplies from health-food shops and by mail order. There is also something extremely satisfying about going into your garden to collect a few sprigs of lemon balm to make a relaxing tea when you feel stressed or getting your own back on the rampant chickweed by putting it to good use as a healing ointment.

Making herbal medicines is not only satisfying, it is also extremely low cost – and just because home-grown products are virtually free, it doesn't make them any less effective.

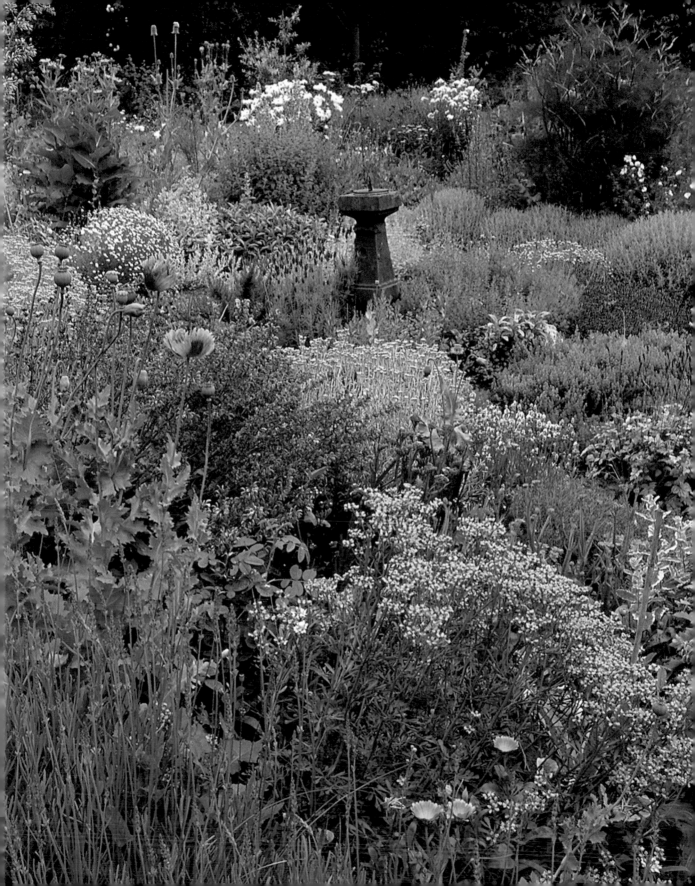

a **medicinal** herb **garden**

Many common garden flowers are actually potent medicinal plants, so the label "herb garden" can cover a multitude of specimens. Lily of the valley (*Convallaria majalis*), for example, is used by professional herbalists to treat heart problems, while in Chinese medicine decorative shrubs also have their uses: buddleia (*Buddleja davidii*) provides a remedy for cataracts and forsythia (*Forsythia suspensa*) is a favourite to clear infections. Many of the wildflower healers listed in Part 2 – such as shepherd's purse, dandelion and cleavers – can usually be found lurking in weedy corners. Although many commonly grown culinary herbs, such as sage, thyme and parsley, are also useful medicinally, some of the more valuable therapeutic plants are unlikely to be grown in a basic herb garden, so it is well worth sowing some native wild flowers like St John's wort, agrimony and wood betony.

Many of the plants discussed in detail in **Part 2** are ideal to grow at home. Others that can deserve a place in the medicinal herb garden include:

Lady's mantle (*Alchemilla vulgaris*) – the aerial parts are useful as a menstrual regulator and styptic. The dew which collects in lady's mantle leaves was once thought to contain magical properties

Heartsease or wild pansy (*Viola tricolor*) – ideal for a variety of skin conditions and inflammations, including nappy rash, heartsease is also used internally for coughs and chest problems. Use the aerial parts.

Marjoram (*Origanum vulgare*) is usually regarded as a culinary herb but is also a tonic remedy, soothing the nerves and warming the digestive system: use in teas for period cramps and headaches.

Melilot or king's clover (*Melilotus officinalis*) is an excellent remedy for varicose veins and eczema. The plant is tall with bright yellow flowers. Collect while flowering and use in creams and washes.

Growing herbs

Home-grown and freshly dried herbs tend to be far more potent than commercial specimens which may have been stored for many months before sale. Growing herbs is also no more difficult than cultivating any other sorts of herbaceous plants or shrubs, while garden herbs provide a constant array of healing aromas to enjoy.

Herbs can prove attractive, too: variegated varieties generally have only slightly less therapeutic properties than basic species and are usually less vigorous, so may be preferable if space is limited. For the less common medicinal herbs, home cultivation can also ensure a constant supply. Obviously, chemical pesticides should be avoided for any herbs intended for medicinal use.

Buying plants

As always when buying nursery-grown plants, look for strong, healthy specimens with plenty of new growth and space in the pot for expansion. Straggly, yellowing herbs will not improve when planted out in the garden – they'll simply be a disappointment.

Although it is especially satisfying to watch your herbs grow from seeds, some species are slow growing or difficult to propagate, so are worth buying as plants to help establish the herb garden. If you want the more decorative varieties of herbs then a visit to a good specialist nursery is essential: worth looking for are variegated lemon balm, variegated mugwort, red ribwort plantain and the various pink-, white- and blue-flowered versions of hyssop, lavender and rosemary.

Most specialist herb nurseries expect a peak in sales in mid- to late spring and will gear production to these times. Later in the season plants are likely to become pot bound with a mass of tangled roots emerging at the bottom and sometimes numerous annual weeds sharing the pot. Good nurseries will regularly pot up their products to larger containers as the season progresses, but then the price usually rises accordingly.

When buying plants always examine them closely for any pests: red spider mite, aphids and whitefly can congregate on the underside of leaves or on new growth and will prove unwelcome additions to a healthy garden. You can check on roots and potting practices by upturning the pot and tapping gently so that plant and compost slide out of the container. Healthy root growth should be evident and the compost should hold its shape. Loose soil suggests that the plant has only recently been potted up and there has been little time to establish the root system.

Always check that plants are correctly labelled: garden centres and even specialist nurseries do not always get names quite right and plant tags can be misplaced. Try to have a little idea of what the plant should look like before buying or ask nursery staff to check if you are unsure.

Herbs mentioned in this book which are worth buying as established plants include: agrimony, comfrey, fennel, hyssop, lavender, lemon balm, marshmallow, meadowsweet, peppermint, rosemary, purple sage, skullcap, thyme, wood betony and yarrow

Growing from seed

It is never worth buying annual herbs in pots – as with garden flowers, they are far better grown from seed, ideally planted directly in the garden where they will spend the summer. The patient can cultivate their own perennial medicinal herbs from seed, too, although generally taking cuttings or dividing established plants is quicker, more efficient and avoids any hybridisation. Seeds for common herbs are often sold alongside vegetable seeds in garden centres, although many medicinal herbs (including toadflax and wood betony) are more likely to be found in the wild flower sections.

Many herbs will self-seed enthusiastically, which can be both a useful source of new plants and a nuisance demanding ruthless weeding out. Particular culprits can include fennel, feverfew, lemon balm and skullcap.

Annual medicinal herbs to sow regularly include borage, Californian poppy, German chamomile and marigold. Sow annual seeds where they are intended to grow once the soil is warm enough.

Perennial herbs easy to grow from seed include coltsfoot, elecampane, fennel, feverfew, hyssop, green sage, wood betony, wild thyme, hops, St John's wort, ribwort plantain and skullcap. Sow biennial or perennial seeds in a seed tray or 7.5 cm pot containing well-watered, good-quality compost. Cover larger seeds with a fine layer of compost roughly equal in depth to the size of the seed, but leave small seeds uncovered. Cover the tray with glass or place the pot in a plastic bag and store in a warm place (up to about 20°C). Alternatively, use a heated propagator.

As soon as the seedlings are large enough to handle prick them out into a second seed tray, eventually potting on into 7.5-10 cm pots before hardening off and planting out. Most seeds should be sown in spring, although perennials are often best sown in late summer or early autumn. Pot these on, over-winter in a greenhouse or cold frame and plant them out the following spring.

Growing from cuttings

Woody perennial herbs are best propagated by cuttings rather than grown from seed. Select cuttings from the side shoots of bushy herbs like sage and rosemary, using semi-ripe sprigs, in late summer or early autumn, or choose the new softwood growth in spring and early summer when roots need to develop quickly if the cutting is to survive. Semi-ripe cuttings are usually more successful for medicinal herbs like elder, hyssop, lavender, rosemary, purple sage and thyme.

Simply break or cut off suitable shoots, keeping a heel of the main stem attached if possible. Dip the base of the cutting into hormone rooting powder and set half a dozen cuttings in good-quality compost in a 10 cm pot. Water well. After a few weeks roots should appear at the base of the pot.

Pot on the rooted cuttings into individual 7.5-10 cm pots ready for hardening off and planting out.

Root division

Herbs can also be propagated by root division. Use a small fork to lever clumps of ramsons, for example, apart or divide large roots with a sharp spade in the early spring when growth has just started. Replant immediately after division and water thoroughly. Roman chamomile, peppermint and elecampane can be propagated by taking the small offsets and runners they develop and replanting.

Keeping them under control

Herbs can grow rapidly and need vigorous pruning to keep in check. For medicinal herb cultivation, regular cropping usually limits the need to do too much pruning. If you cut herbaceous herbs back to 10-15 cm when collecting aerial parts for drying that is usually all that is needed. Where specific parts of a plant are used (e.g. lavender flowers), then normal gardening rules for pruning apply.

Prune shrubby herbs like rosemary, sage and lavender (after flowering) in late summer, cutting back to leave around 10-20 cm of the new growth.

A healthy window box

Herbs will grow happily for one or two seasons in containers or window boxes, although fresh planting each spring will ensure healthier plants and a better balance in sizes. Remember, too, that herbs thrive in poor soil, so rich potting compost can encourage excess growth. Use a loam-based compost or add one part of grit to five parts of peat-based compost to improve the soil texture and drainage.

Suitable plants for a medicinal herbal window box include: variegated lemon balm, Roman chamomile, wood betony, creeping thyme (*Thymus serpyllum*), a small sage plant, nasturtiums (*Tropaeolum majus*) which are bitter, diuretic and antiseptic – ideal for urinary infections and wounds, and variegated ground ivy (*Glechoma hederacea*) – a useful anti-catarrhal for colds and running noses.

Harvesting herbs

The time when herbs are gathered can significantly affect the constituent chemicals and thus the therapeutic properties. In the past complex rituals were followed so that herbs were gathered when they were at their most potent; old herbals often give detailed instructions as to when to gather plants – at what time of day, phase of the moon or in which sign of the zodiac.

Today, many of these traditions appear bizarre and groundless, but often they did in fact pinpoint the time when the herb was at its peak. Vervain, for example, was gathered when the dog star, Sirius, could be seen in the heavens (around 11 August), which – in the northern hemisphere – is generally a time when it is coming into flower and is probably at its best.

Harvesting traditions such as these survive most obviously today in Tibetan medicine, in which herbs are often collected at times that are astrologically significant for the individual patient. The practitioner will study the history of the disease, the precise time of onset and so on, and will then choose the correct time to collect the remedy in this particular case.

For Western herb gatherers, however, more prosaic considerations include collecting the herbs on a dry day, when the plants are at the peak of maturity and thus when the concentration of active ingredients is highest.

Flowers

These should be collected when fully open and handled carefully as they are easily damaged. Small flowers like lavender can be dried on their stems but if the stem is fleshy – like mullein (*Verbascum thapsis*) – the flowers must be removed and dried individually. An easy way to dry individual flowers is to spread them on trays and place in an airing cupboard for a couple of days.

Leaves

Large leaves (such as burdock) can be gathered individually, but smaller ones (like lemon balm) are best left on the stem. Leaves of deciduous herbs should generally be gathered just before flowering; evergreen ones like rosemary can be collected throughout the

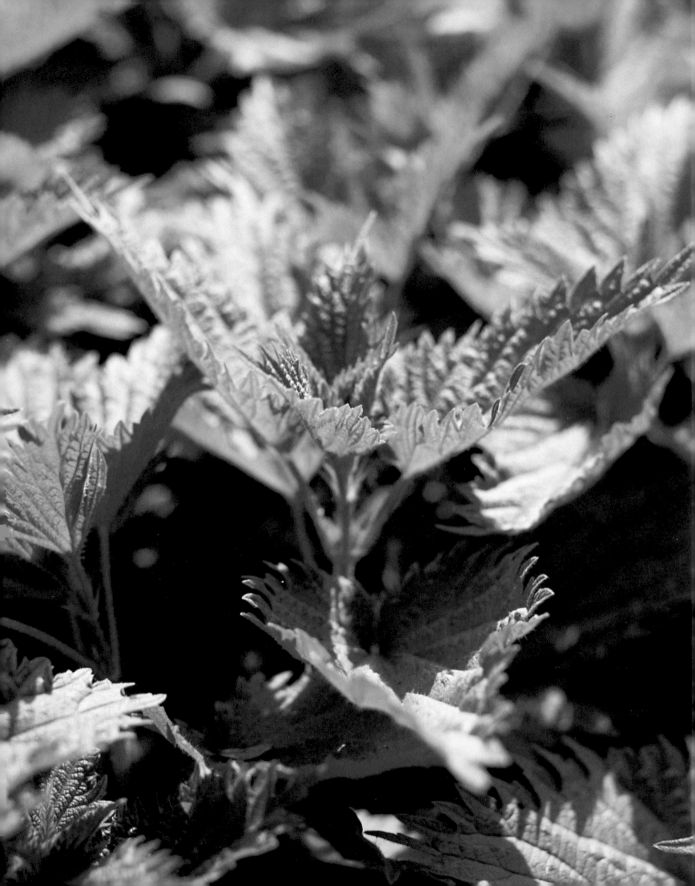

year. Sometimes young leaves are picked early in the season for cooking or spring tonics (such as stinging nettles or dandelions for soups and salads). A second crop of the more mature leaves can then be taken closer to flowering time. Coltsfoot and butterbur leaves appear after the flowers so should be gathered then.

Aerial parts

If you are using all the aerial parts then the best time to collect is in the midst of flowering, giving a mixture of leaves, stem, flowers and seed-head. Skullcap, for example, can be collected when around half the flowers have formed the characteristic cap-shaped pod.

Seeds

These should be collected when ripe. For plants with large seed-heads like fennel, it is best to gather them when around two-thirds of the seeds on a particular head are ripe and before too many have been dispersed by the wind or taken by birds.

Fruit

Berries and other fruits should be gathered when just ripe, before the fruit becomes too soft or pulpy to dry effectively.

Roots

Roots are generally gathered in the autumn when the aerial parts of the plant have died down and before the ground becomes too hard to make digging difficult. An exception is dandelion, whose roots should be gathered in spring when the carbohydrate content of the root is at its lowest and the concentration of medicinal constituents is thus greater.

Bark

This is generally best collected in the autumn, when the sap is falling, to minimise damage to the plant. Never remove all the bark – or a band of bark completely surrounding a tree – unless you really do want to sacrifice the plant to herbal medicine.

Saps and resin

These can be collected from trees by making a deep incision in the bark in autumn when the sap is falling. In most cases a cup attached to the tree will be an adequate receptacle, but sometimes a large bucket may be needed: a substantial amount of birch sap, for example, can be collected overnight at certain times of year. Aloe gel can be obtained by splitting the leaf open and scraping the thick gelatinous sap into a bowl using the blunt side of a knife. Latex from plants like wild lettuce and greater celandine can be extracted by squeezing the leaf stems over a bowl. Many saps can be corrosive, so protective gloves should be worn. Saps can generally be stored for a few days in a refrigerator or can be preserved by boiling to form a reduced paste.

Bulbs and corms

These should be gathered after the aerial parts have died down. Collect garlic corms quickly as they tend to move downwards in the soil once the leaves have wilted and can be difficult to find.

Drying herbs

Herbs need to be dried as quickly as possible and away from bright sunlight to preserve the aromatic ingredients and prevent oxidation of other chemicals. A good circulation of air is also needed, so tie stems in small bunches and leave the airing cupboard door slightly ajar when drying petals. A dry garden shed with a low-powered fan heater running can be effective, but avoid drying herbs in garages as they can become contaminated with petrol fumes. In warm conditions with a good circulation of air it is possible to dry herbs completely within five or six days, sometimes even less. The longer the plant takes to dry the more likely it is to discolour and lose its flavour. Ideally the temperature in the drying room should be between 20-32°C/70-90°F and should never go above 38°C/100°F.

With experience it is possible to know precisely when the herbs are dry enough to bottle. They should be crumbled gently and stored in clean dry jars or pots with air-tight lids. If the herbs are stored when still slightly damp they will go mouldy. Jars should ideally be of coloured glass or pottery or kept out of direct sunlight which speeds deterioration. Do not store herbs in metal or plastic containers.

Some people use a microwave oven for drying herbs but recent research work has shown that such radiation can cause changes to the complex chemicals in herbs with entirely new substances, of unknown toxicity or efficacy, being produced in the process. It is therefore best to avoid this technique for medicinal herbs.

Some herbs freeze well – especially fennel, dill, parsley and basil. They can be chopped and frozen in ice cube trays or wrapped in plastic film in small bunches. This is ideal for culinary use but the sort of quantities needed for medicinal applications generally makes freezing impractical.

Remember to label dried herbs with the variety, source and date. If dried and stored properly, most will keep for 12-18 months without significant deterioration.

However, there are exceptions: valerian and hops both change their chemical composition over time, so the action of the herb can vary with age.

Flowers
Collect the flowers on a dry day when the morning dew has evaporated and remove obvious dirt, grit, insects, etc. Then spread the flower heads on newspaper or trays and place in the airing cupboard or in a warm spare room to dry. Lavender flowers are best treated like seeds and dried in bunches covered with a loosely tied paper bag. Small flowers can be left intact but marigold petals are best pulled from the flower heads when dried and the central part of the flower discarded. Store in dark glass/pottery containers or in cupboards.

Leaves/Aerial parts
Collect on a dry day and tie in small bunches of about five to eight stems which can be hung in a garden shed, spare room or other dry, airy, warm place. When the leaves are brittle, but not so dry that they turn to powder when touched, the herb is ready. Always dry leafy herbs while still on the stem. Once dried, the leaves can easily be rubbed from the stem and the larger pieces discarded. If you are using the entire aerial parts of a plant, then flowers, stem, seed heads and leaves can be crumbled together before storing.

Seeds
Collect entire seed heads with about 15-25 cm of stalk when the seeds are almost ripe and hang them in small bunches loosely covered with paper bags, away from direct sunlight. The seeds will fall off when they are ripe

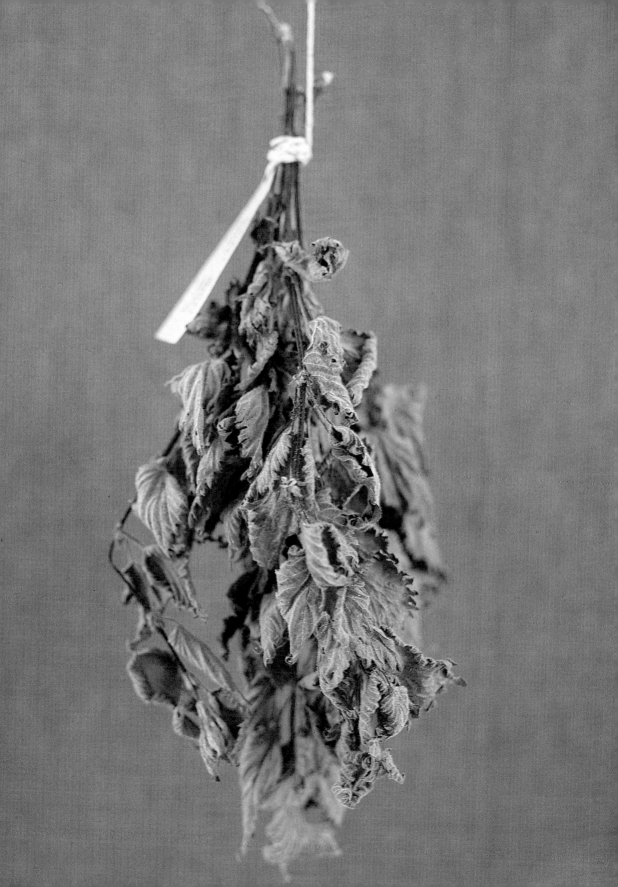

and will be collected in the bag during the following couple of weeks.

Berries

These should be picked when just ripe and spread on trays in an airing cupboard. Fleshy fruits should be turned regularly to ensure even drying and any with signs of mould discarded.

Roots

Wash roots thoroughly to remove soil and dirt. It is best to chop large roots into small pieces when still fresh as they can be difficult to cut when dry. Spread the pieces on trays and dry for two to three hours in a cooling oven (i.e. an oven with no direct heat). Repeat this process for large roots, then transfer to an airing cupboard or quiet sunny room to complete drying undisturbed. Roots need to be stored in dry, air-tight containers away from sunlight. Some tend to reabsorb moisture from the air and should be discarded if they become soft.

Bark

Dust or wipe bark to remove moss or insects – avoid soaking in water too much. Then break into manageable pieces (1-3 cm square) and spread on trays in an airing cupboard or warm, dry, airy room.

Buying dried herbs

For those with limited growing space, there is now – fortunately – a good choice of suppliers of dried herb both in high-street shops and by mail order (see page 188). Always buy in small quantities (250-500 g) to avoid unnecessary home storage and where possible

examine material before buying to check on quality. Choose herbs which have a good colour and aroma and are not faded or musty-smelling.

Avoid shops which display herbs in clear glass jars on sunny shelves – the quality will probably be disappointing. Poor storage can lead to rapid deterioration with mouse droppings, mould and insects among unwanted pollutants.

Ideally buy organic herbs or those labelled as "wild crafted", which means they have been collected in the wild rather than grown as a commercial – and often heavily sprayed – cash crop. Poor harvesting can lead to many unwanted additions – dried grass, for example, is often found with herbs which have been gathered from meadow areas. With practice one soon learns to recognise the characteristics of many dried herbs so it becomes easier to check on the accuracy of labels. Skullcap, for example, has characteristic seed pods, agrimony has small burrs and many herbs can be identified from their aroma.

Mistakes can and do happen, however. A classic error was confusion over wood sage (*Teucrium scorodonia*) and skullcap which for many years led to a description of wood sage being included in herbals under skullcap. Another well-documented error concerned the supplier who sold sea mayweed (*Matricaria maritima*) as feverfew – the plants are similar in appearance but the mayweed lacks feverfew's therapeutic constituents, so would be useless for treating migraine.

Making and buying remedies

There are many ways to use herbs – both internally and externally. Some techniques are quick and easy, such as making teas; others require preparation: it can take at least two weeks to prepare a tincture, so this is not a method to use if you need medication in a hurry. Ointments and creams also take time and practice, although it is not difficult to make good-quality products with a little experience. Remember also that herbs vary in quality, character and moisture content throughout the year, so that at some times a good yield of juice is available or you may need to add less liquid to creams made from fresh herbs.

Having mastered the basic production skills the next problem is deciding which herbs to use: they can, of course, be used individually – as simples – and will often prove very effective. However, herbs generally work best in combinations. Some herbalists will limit their mixtures to four or five herbs, others may include up to 20 in a single prescription. In traditional Chinese medicine, practitioners use classic formulae for particular syndromes. These prescriptions have often been unchanged for hundreds of years and all students of traditional Chinese medicine have to learn many hundreds of recipes by heart before qualifying.

For home use it is best to keep combinations as simple as possible, limiting mixtures to two or three well-chosen herbs. As combining a few grams of herbs for a day's dosages can be complicated, use around 25-30 g of each chosen herb, shake the dried herbs together thoroughly and store in a clean, dry jar. It is then easy to measure out 25 g of the combination to make the day's dose of infusion as required.

One can mix equal amounts of herbs or use more of whichever one seems most appropriate for the current health problem. A cough made worse by catarrh, for example, could be treated by coltsfoot flowers (15 g) with elder flowers (5 g) and hyssop (5 g), or a tension headache may respond to a combination of relaxing herbs (skullcap, 10 g) with some which are more closely targeted at headaches (7.5 g, each of wood betony and lavender flowers, perhaps). Suggestions for combining herbs are given in Part 3 of this book.

It can also be useful to combine external and internal remedies. Rosemary oil, used topically, for example, can bring fast relief for arthritic pains while devil's claw taken internally may need four or six weeks to start controlling the problem.

Infusions

An infusion is simply a tea made by steeping the herb in freshly boiled water for 10 minutes. Traditionally 1 oz (25 g) of dried herb was used to 1 pint (500 ml) of boiled water, which is sufficient for three doses, and the method can be used for most leafy herbs and flowers. The herb needs to be put into a ceramic or glass teapot or jug (with lid) and it is important for the water to go just off the boil, otherwise many aromatic plant constituents will be lost in the excessive steam. After infusing, strain through a sieve – as with conventional tea leaves – and take a wine-glass dose (about 150 ml) three times a day. Sweeten with a little honey if required. If using fresh herb you need three times as much to allow for the additional weight of water in fresh plant material i.e. 75 g to 500 ml of water.

The infusion can be reheated before each dose – this is helpful if the tea is being used for a "cold" condition, such as chills or arthritis, although in many cases it can be drunk cold as well. It is best to make only enough infusion for one day's doses, although surplus can be stored in a refrigerator for up to 48 hours.

Herbs listed in this book which can be made into infusions include:

agrimony, bear's breech, bilberry, birch leaves, borage, buchu, burdock, Californian poppy, celery, chamomile, chickweed, cleavers, coffee, coltsfoot, common mallow, cornflower, creeping Jenny, daisy, dandelion leaves, echinacea leaves, elder flowers, fennel, feverfew, ginkgo, grape, greater celandine, hawthorn, herb Robert, hops, hyssop, isphaghula, Jack by the hedge, lavender, lemon balm, linden, marigold, marsh woundwort, marshmallow, meadowsweet, olive, passion flower, peppermint, plantain, purple loosestrife, raspberry, rosemary, sage, self-heal, shepherd's purse, skullcap, St John's wort, stinging nettle, strawberries, tea, thyme, toadflax, vervain, white deadnettle, witch hazel, wood avens, wood betony and yarrow

China decoctions are always used instead of infusions with as much as 100 g (4 oz) or more of dried herbs heated in 500-1000 ml (1–2 pt) of water.

Decoctions can be reduced down to 100-250 ml with further heating and then this mix can be used in drop dosages either neat or in water. This can be a good way to administer decoctions to children who are often reluctant to drink whole cups of herbal brews.

Herbs listed in this book which can be made into decoctions include:

birch, bitter orange, burdock root, butterbur, cinnamon, cloves, daisy, dandelion root, devil's claw, echinacea root, elder bark and root, elecampane, ginger, ginseng, golden seal, lettuce, liquorice, Siberian ginseng, slippery elm, witch hazel and yellow dock.

Decoctions

A decoction is like a tea, but it is made by simmering the plant material for 15-20 minutes and is ideal for tougher plant components like bark, roots and berries, where it can be more difficult to extract the active ingredients.

Traditionally one used 1 oz (25 g) of herb to 1½ pint (750 ml) of cold water, which should then be brought to the boil in a stainless steel, glass, ceramic or enamel saucepan (not aluminium) and allowed to simmer until the volume has been reduced by about a third.

The mixture is then treated as an infusion: strained through a sieve and taken in three wine-glass doses during the day. As with infusions, the tea can be warmed through before each dose and sweetened with a little honey as required, and it is best to make only enough for one day's doses at a time, although surplus can be stored in a refrigerator for up to 48 hours. In

Macerations

Although most roots can be made into decoctions, some respond better to cold maceration which helps to preserve many active constituents which tend to be broken down by heating. Simply put 25 g of the chopped root into a teapot or basin, cover with 500 ml of cold water and leave overnight. Next day, strain the mixture through a sieve and use in three wine-glass doses during the day or as required.

As with decoctions and infusions, macerations are best prepared on a daily basis, although they can be stored in a refrigerator for up to 48 hours. This method is ideal for marshmallow and valerian roots.

Combined infusions and decoctions

When using a number of herbs in a tea it is often necessary to use some as infusions and some as

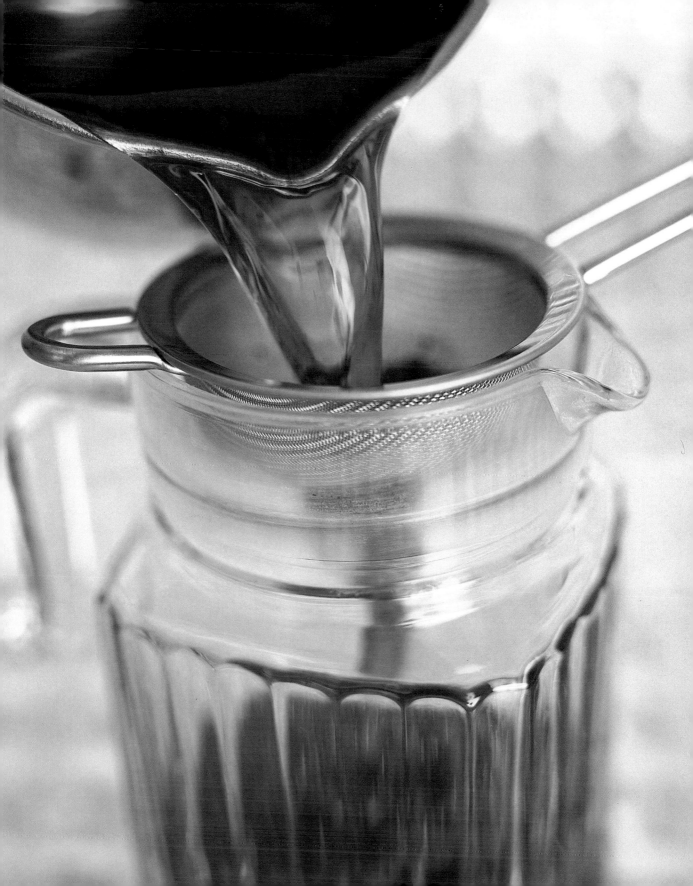

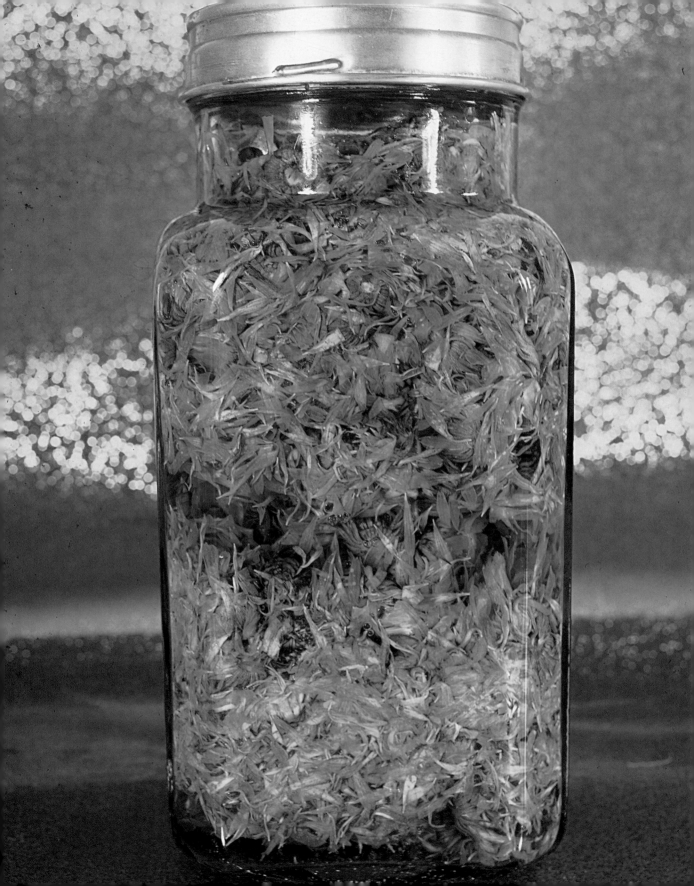

decoctions – for example, if one were making a tea of yellow dock root with burdock leaves for skin problems. In these cases, measure out 750 ml of water and use this to simmer the required amount of roots (perhaps 10 or 15 g). Once the volume has reduced by about a third, pour the still simmering mixture over the dried herb, in a jug, and infuse for a further 10-15 minutes.

The tea can then be used as for simple infusions or decoctions (see above).

Tinctures

A tincture is an alcoholic extraction of the active ingredients in a herb made by soaking the dried or fresh plant material in a mixture of alcohol and water.

Commercially produced tinctures are usually made from ethyl alcohol with the supply of duty-free alcohol strictly controlled in many countries by the Customs and Excise authorities. Commercially made tinctures can sometimes be extremely expensive since, in Britain, the customs officials regard the more pleasant-tasting tinctures – including those made from aniseed, caraway, cinnamon, lavender, lemon balm, orange peel and rosemary – as being in the liqueur category and thus liable to duty.

Although any alcohol can be used to make tinctures, not all alcohols are safe to drink, so great care needs to be taken with home production. Methyl alcohol is extremely poisonous and, although some herbalists have used isopropyl alcohol (rubbing alcohol) for tincture-making, this too can be very toxic. Glycerol has the benefit of being very low cost, and is ideal for children and others who should avoid alcohol, but the resulting tinctures are slightly slimy to the taste. For home use, probably the safest and most accessible source of alcohol is in the drinks cabinet – in the form of spirits and wines.

Most tinctures are made from a mixture containing 25% alcohol in water (i.e. 25 ml of pure alcohol with 75 ml of water). This is slightly weaker in strength than most proof spirits – vodka, whisky, rum, gin etc – so a suitable mixture can easily be made by diluting over-the-counter drinks. Of commonly available spirits, vodka is generally considered the most appropriate as it has fewer other flavourings or herbal ingredients. Using rum is a good way to disguise the less palatable herbs. For a standard 25% alcohol mixture simply add a further 500 ml of water to a 1 litre bottle of vodka (37.5% alcohol) to make 1500 ml of a 25% alcohol/water mixture that can then be used for tincture making.

Standard tinctures are usually made in the weight:volume proportion 1:5 (i.e. 1 kg of herb to 5 litres of alcohol/water mixture or 1 lb of herb to 5 pt of liquid). For domestic use mixing 200 g of herb with 1 litre of liquid usually produces a sufficient quantity to make at any one time. With fresh herb, you need three times as much to account for the water content of the herb (i.e. 600 g of fresh herb to 1 litre of liquid). Some herbs – mainly roots, barks or those which contain a lot of resins or essential oils – need to be extracted in 45-60% alcohol mixtures. This is more difficult to obtain for domestic use. Using 25% alcohol will give a slightly weaker product compared with commercial tinctures, although if using home-grown herbs their freshness will more than make up for any loss of potency.

To make a tincture simply put the required quantity of herb into a large jar (ideally an old-fashioned glass screw-top sweet jar). Shake thoroughly, then cover with the alcohol/water mixture and store in a cool place for two weeks, shaking the mixture occasionally. Strain the mixture through a wine press or jelly bag and store the resulting liquid in clean, dark glass containers. The herbal residue is an ideal addition to the compost heap.

Tinctures will generally last for two years or more without deterioration – although Ayurvedic medicine actually argues that the tinctures increase in potency as they age.

Fluid extracts

More concentrated alcohol/water extracts are available commercially as "fluid extracts", although these can be more complex to make at home. The herb to liquid ratio is around 1:1 and they are generally made by macerating the herb in five times its weight of liquid (as for a tincture) for up to two weeks and then heating the mix in a percolator to reduce the volume to around a half. This liquid is collected and reserved. Fresh alcohol/water is then added to the mixture and the cycle of maceration and percolating repeated twice more. Eventually the various extracts are combined.

Because the alcohol will have evaporated during the process, fluid extracts do not last as long as tinctures and often need to have extra alcohol added for long-term storage. Fluid extracts are, by definition, five times stronger than the average 1:5 tincture, so need be used only in very small quantities. If the dose of a tincture is 5 ml, then 1 ml of a fluid extract will deliver the same amount of herb.

Professional herbalists often use fluid extracts when large amounts of a herb are needed: dandelion leaf, for example, used as a diuretic is often given in the form of a fluid extract.

Tonic wines

Tincture-like extracts can be made with wine, although they tend not to keep so well. Steeping the herb in wine was a traditional way of making medicines in the past and many early herbals mention this method. It is also a good way to make tonics – simply put a large quantity of herb in a vinegar vat (available from cook shops) and cover with a good-quality red wine to make a wonderful healing brew for regular use. The Chinese tonic herbs, such as Korean ginseng and *Dang Gui* work well in this method, as does elecampane root. It is important to keep the herb covered with wine, otherwise the plant material is likely to go mouldy.

Traditional flower wines can also be made in this way. Simply gather healing petals as they appear through the year – start with coltsfoot, violet (*Viola odorata*), primroses (*Primula vulgaris*) and cowslips (*Primula veris*), and add honeysuckle (*Lonicera japonica*), heartsease (*Viola tricolor*), St John's wort, roses (*Rosa* spp.), mullein (*Verbascum thapsus*), hollyhock, mallow and wood betony as the summer progresses. Put the fresh flowers into a vinegar vat and cover each layer of petals with more wine. By the end of the year the vat will be filled and the liquid can be run off to make a revitalising drink for cold winter days. Tonic wines can be delicious – but limit intake to a small wine glass (about 75 ml) a day!

Juices

Processing a herb through a liquidiser is an easy way to make a juice of the entire plant, rather than trying to extract constituents by water or alcohol. The method is ideal for soft, leafy plants – such as cleavers, lemon balm, St John's wort or fennel – and can also be used for fruits and vegetables.

Typical dosage for a juice is 10 ml (a dessertspoon) three times a day. The juice will last only for a few days in a refrigerator and soon deteriorates, so it is best to make small quantities (100 ml or so) at a time.

Commercial juices are available from many suppliers and it is, of course, very easy to find carrot, tomato or beetroot juice in supermarkets.

Of the plants mentioned in this book, juices available over-the-counter include:

artichoke, asparagus, beetroot, birch, borage, cabbage, carrot, celery, chamomile, coltsfoot, dandelion, echinacea, fennel, fig, garlic, hawthorn, horseradish, juniper, lemon balm, oats, onion, potato, ramsons, rosemary, sage, St John's wort, stinging nettle, thyme, tomato, valerian, watercress and yarrow.

Syrups

Sugar or honey can be used to preserve herbal infusions and decoctions and are ideal for cough remedies as the sweetness is also soothing.

Syrups are easy to produce at home by using a standard infusion or decoction (depending on the type of herb to be used). After straining the mixture make a syrup by adding 500 ml of liquid to 500 g of unrefined sugar or honey. Heat the mixture in a cast iron or stainless steel saucepan, stirring constantly to dissolve the sugar or honey and make a syrup. Allow the mixture

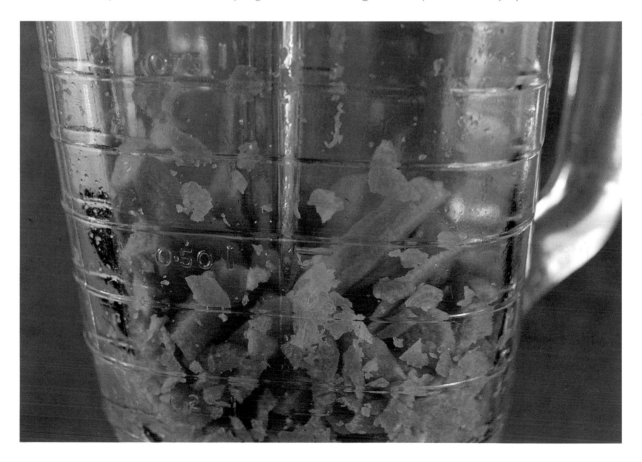

to cool and store in clean glass bottles with a cork, not a screw top – the cork is important, as syrups often ferment and tight screw tops can easily cause exploding bottles.

Useful plants for cough syrups include

coltsfoot, elecampane, hyssop, lemon, liquorice, marshmallow, onion, ribwort plantain and thyme.

Ointments and creams

Creams are a mixture of oils or fats and water and are described as being miscible (meaning that they mix in with or can be absorbed by the skin), while ointments contain only oils or fats and form a separate layer over the skin. Ointments are suitable where the skin is already weak or soft or where some protection from additional moisture is needed (as in ointments for nappy rash). Traditionally, ointments were made using animal fats and the simplest method is to heat dried herbs in melted lard or Vaseline for a couple of hours.

Creams can easily be made using emulsifying ointment (available from most pharmacists). This is a mixture of oils (usually hydrocarbons or paraffins) which can be blended with a certain proportion of water to make a cream. The usual production method involves heating the dried herb in a mixture of emulsifying ointment and water (or a water/alcohol mixture for better extraction of the herb's active ingredients). Typical proportions with this method are: 300 g emulsifying ointment, 135 ml glycerol, 165 ml water and 60 g dried herb.

An alternative to emulsifying ointment is to use: 100 g sunflower oil (or similar), 25 g white beeswax, 25 g anhydrous lanolin, 75 ml of water, 25 ml glycerol and 50 g dried herb. In either case the basic method is to melt the emulsifying ointment or fats in a double saucepan over water. Then add the rest of the ingredients and heat for three hours. Press the mixture through a fine nylon sieve, jelly bag or wine press and then stir the cream constantly until it is cold before storing in clean, air-tight plastic or glass jars. Creams made in this way will usually keep for several months, although their shelf life can be prolonged by storing in a cool larder or refrigerator or by adding five drops of benzoin (sold amongst aromatherapy oils or in pharmacies) to the mixture as a preservative.

This method is suitable for making creams of:

marigold petals, comfrey herb or root, chickweed herb, cleavers herb, lemon balm herb, St John's wort flowering tops, chamomile flowers or stinging nettles.

Infused oils

Infused oils can be used in making ointments or as a base for massage oils and are an excellent and simple way of creating external herbal remedies. There are two techniques: hot infusion or cold infusion.

Hot infusion

These are made by heating 100 g of dried (300 g of fresh) herb in 500 ml of sunflower oil (or similar) in a double saucepan over water for about three hours. Remember to refill the lower saucepan with hot water from time to time to prevent it from boiling dry. After about three hours the oil will take on a greenish colour and it can then be strained and squeezed through a muslin bag or wine press and stored in clean glass bottles, away from direct sunlight.

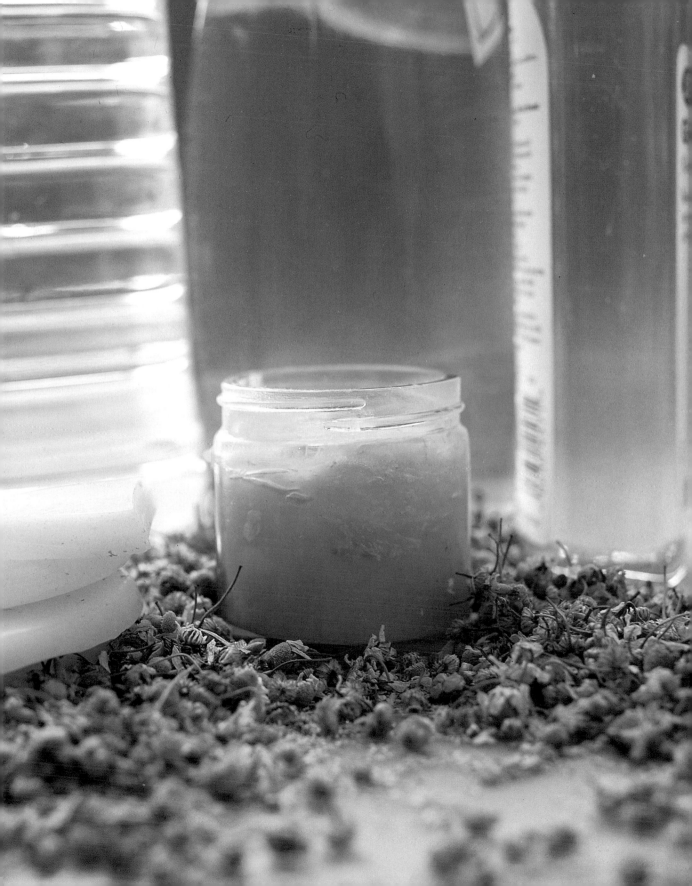

This method is suitable for making oils of:

comfrey, chickweed, stinging nettle or infused rosemary oil.

Cold infusion

Because the oil is not heated in this method, one can use good-quality seed oils that are rich in essential fatty acids (EFAs) – such as *gamma*-linolenic or *cis*-linoleic – which have significant therapeutic properties. Oils high in EFAs include walnut, safflower and pumpkin oils. The infused oil is made by simply filling a large jar with the dried or fresh herb and completely covering with oil. The jar should be left on a sunny windowsill or in the greenhouse for at least three weeks; then the mixture can be strained through a wine press or jelly bag. Ideally the whole process should then be repeated using fresh herb and the once-infused oil – again leaving it in a sunny place for a further two or three weeks. Finally, the oil can be strained and stored in clean, air-tight bottles.

The cold infused method is suitable for:

St John's wort, marigold or chamomile flowers.

These infused oils – which will generally last for at least a year, often longer – can be thickened with beeswax and anhydrous lanolin (which you can order through your pharmacist) to make ointments or with a mixture of beeswax, lanolin and herbal tincture to make creams.

Ointment: use 100 ml of infused oil, 25 g beeswax, 25 g anhydrous lanolin. Melt the fats in a double saucepan and add the infused oil. Pour into clean glass jars while still warm and allow to cool.

Cream: use 100 ml infused oil, 25 g beeswax, 25 g

anhydrous lanolin and 50 ml herbal tincture. Melt the wax and lanolin in a double saucepan and add the infused oil. Remove from the heat and pour in the tincture, stirring constantly. The cream forms as the mixture cools and can be spooned into small, clean glass jars for storage. Various combination creams using different oil and herb/tincture mixtures are easy to make: try comfrey and rosemary for arthritic pain or chamomile and St John's wort for inflammations.

Massage oils

The sort of massage oils used in aromatherapy are very easy to make at home by adding a few drops of essential oil to some sort of oil base. Suitable bases include sweet almond oil, wheatgerm oil, avocado oil or any of the infused herb oils made from walnut or sunflower oil described above.

Essential oils are made commercially, usually by steam-distilling various parts of the plant. This is not a technique for home use.

In general do not use more than 10% of essential oil (10 drops of essential oil in a teaspoon or 5 ml of carrier oil), as many essential oils can irritate sensitive skins. Always buy good-quality essential oils as many cheap ones are chemically adulterated. The higher the price and the more reputable the brand name, the more likely the oil is to be good quality.

Try some of these relaxing massage combinations:

Strains and sprains – use 5-10 drops each of rosemary, eucalyptus, juniper and lavender oil in 50 ml of infused comfrey or St John's wort oil.

Arthritis and rheumatism – use 5-10 drops each of

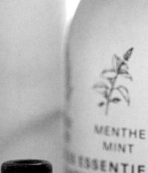

rosemary, lavender, sage and marjoram in 50 ml of infused bladderwrack (*Fucus vesiculosus*) or infused rosemary oil.

Migraine and headaches – use 5 drops each of lavender, marjoram and lemon balm oil in 25 ml of sweet almond or wheatgerm oil.

General relaxing oil – use 5 drops each of basil, sandalwood, lemon balm and lavender in 25 ml of St John's wort or sweet almond oil.

Chest rubs are ideal for treating many respiratory and throat problems, including coughs, bronchitis, whooping cough, laryngitis and asthma. Use 5-10 drops of thyme, hyssop and eucalyptus oil in sweet almond or wheatgerm oil and massage into the chest two or three times a day.

Steam inhalants

Inhaling aromatic oils is a good way to clear the respiratory system of mucus in conditions such as catarrh, sinusitis, bronchitis or asthma. Either infusions or well-diluted essential oils can be used. It is important to stay in a warm room for 30 minutes after treatment to allow the airways time to return to normal.

Use around 500 ml of a standard infusion or add up to 10 drops of essential oil to a bowl of hot water per treatment. Useful inhalant herbs include chamomile, thyme, eucalyptus, hyssop and peppermint. Repeat treatments once or twice a day, inhaling the steam for 10 minutes each time.

Foot baths

Soaking your feet in a hot bath can bring relief to aching feet, ease sprains and stimulate the circulation for those prone to chilblains; it also helps combat the common cold. Suitable essential oils (see under Baths, below) or hot infusions can be used, or you can opt for a traditional mustard bath, using a tablespoonful of powdered mustard to a basin of hot water.

Alternating hot and cold treatments can help reduce bruising and provide emergency relief for badly sprained ankles. Soak the feet or other affected area in a basin of very hot water containing a large quantity of rosemary sprigs or 20 drops of rosemary essential oil for 3-5 minutes and then plunge into a water and ice mixture for 2-3 minutes. Repeat the process for as long as you can bear it.

Baths

Adding essential oils or an infusion to bath water is an excellent way to ease aching limbs, clear stuffy noses or relax after a stressful day. Use 2-5 drops of essential oil neat in the bath water and stir well to disperse the oil. Alternatively add 500 ml of a freshly made infusion. The following oils – readily available from health food shops and chemists – can be helpful:

Aches and pains – rosemary, lavender, eucalyptus, juniper, marjoram.

Anxiety and stress – benzoin, chamomile, cypress, rose geranium, jasmine, lavender, marjoram, lemon balm, rose, sandalwood.

Catarrh – peppermint, eucalyptus, lavender.

Coughs and colds – hyssop, thyme, benzoin, anise, sandalwood, eucalyptus.

Fatigue – basil, lemon balm, rosemary, sage, peppermint.

Headaches – lavender, rose, marjoram.

Period pain – chamomile, cypress, marjoram, lemon balm, rosemary, sandalwood.

Pessaries and suppositories

Pessaries are waxy pellets containing medication which can be inserted in the vagina and will melt at body temperature, delivering the remedy to the site of infection or irritation.

Suppositories are similar, but intended for anal insertion. They are often used where treatments are needed in the lower bowel and the medicines would otherwise be broken down during the digestive process.

Both can be made at home, although the process can be time consuming without a pessary mould (sometimes available from chemists). An ideal base is cocoa butter which melts at body temperature.

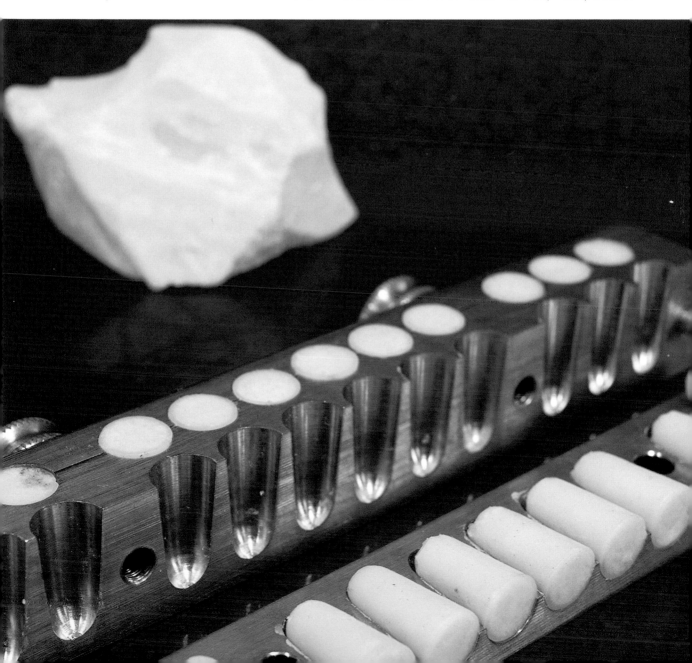

Substitute moulds can be made by shaping cooking foil into small thimble-like holders about 1 cm in diameter and 2 cm long. Melt the cocoa butter in a double saucepan and then add essential oils and pour into the moulds. Twenty grams of cocoa butter with 30 drops of essential oils is generally enough for 24 pessaries. Peel away the cooking foil once the cocoa butter has set and store in a pot lined with greaseproof paper.

Ideally the mould should be lubricated before use, which makes it easier to remove the pessaries. A suitable lubricant can be made from 10 g of soft soap, 50 ml of glycerol and 40 ml of methylated spirit. Shake this together and leave for a couple of days for the soft soap to dissolve thoroughly. Pour this into the mould first, leave for a few seconds, then pour away.

Compresses

Compresses are often used to accelerate healing of wounds or muscle injuries. They are basically cloth pads soaked in herbal extracts and usually applied hot to painful limbs, swellings or strains. Use a clean piece of cotton, cotton wool, linen or surgical gauze soaked in a hot, strained infusion, decoction or tincture (diluted with hot water) and apply to the affected area. When the compress cools repeat using fresh, hot mixture.

Occasionally a cold compress may be used – as with some types of headaches when a cool pad soaked in lavender infusion can be helpful.

Poultices

Poultices have a very similar action to compresses, but involve applying the whole herb to an affected area directly rather than using a liquid extract. Poultices are usually applied hot for swellings, sprains or to draw pus, but cold pastes/poultices can also be useful: apply comfrey root paste to varicose ulcers, for example. As with hot compresses, renew the hot poultice as it cools or place a hot-water bottle on top to keep it hot.

To make a poultice, simply bruise fresh herbs, mix in a food processor for a few seconds or sweat in a pan, then spread the mixture on to gauze and apply to the affected area. If you are using dried herbs or powders, mix them with hot water to make a soft paste, then squeeze out any surplus liquid and spread the residue on gauze or apply directly to the area affected.

If putting poultices directly onto the skin, apply a little vegetable oil first to prevent it from sticking. Poultices are often used to draw splinters or pus from wounds.

Powders and capsules

Although it is possible to grind herbs in a domestic coffee grinder, they usually become very hot in the process and this can cause chemical changes within the plant: grinding hard roots can also damage the coffee grinder! It is best to use powders produced using commercial mills, which do not cause quite so much heating, and many powdered herbs are now available from specialist suppliers.

Two-part gelatine capsules (generally size 00, which holds around 200–250 mg of powder) are available from chemists or specialist health-food shops, although filling them by hand can be a laborious process and it is often easier simply to take an equivalent amount of the powder stirred into a little water instead.

To fill capsules put some herb powder in a saucer or flat dish and then separate the two halves of the capsule. Slide them together through the powder, scooping it into the capsule. Capsule-filling machines are

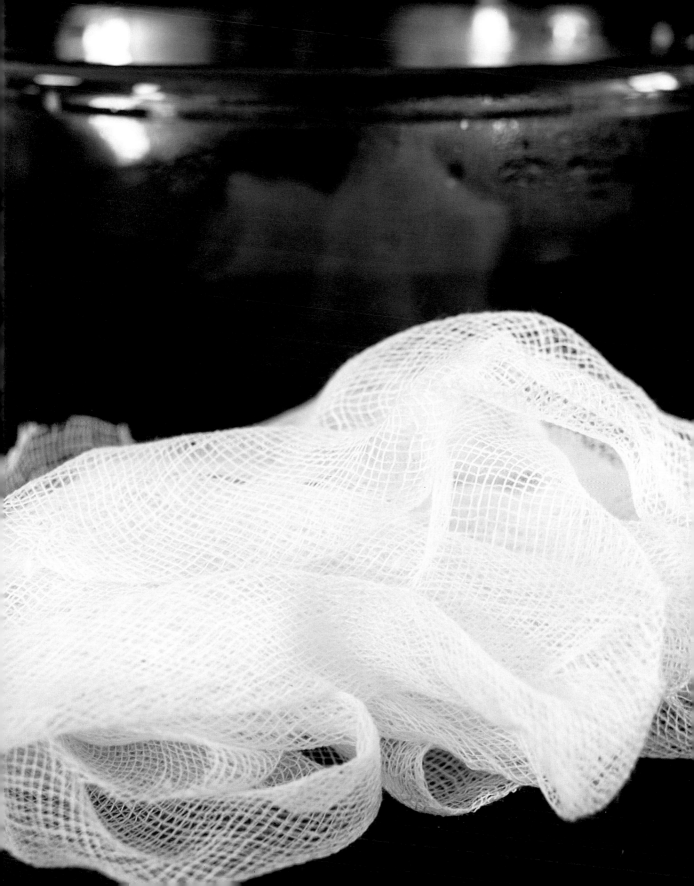

used by many herbalists. These mechanically separate 100 capsules at a time, holding the two halves in plastic frames. Powder is spread over the lower frame, filling the capsules, and then the top frame replaced to reassemble them.

Over-the-counter remedies

Well over 1,000 different herbal remedies can now be found in health-food shops and high-street chemists as retailers capitalise on the growing fashion for herbal products. Many of these are based on traditional remedies devised by herbalists 50 or 100 years ago, while others use more recently discovered herbs or oriental plants that have little history of traditional use within Europe.

Production and distribution of herbal medicines is, quite rightly, strictly regulated in most countries. Despite the popular view that herbs are natural and therefore "safe", many plants are extremely potent and misuse can have serious side effects. In Britain, much of the current legislation stems from the 1968 Thalidomide tragedy when there was an urgent political need to tighten control of both pharmaceutical drugs and herbal medicines. Before then herbal suppliers could make and package what they wanted, often providing helpful names like "Blood Pressure Pills" or "Gall Bladder Remedy" to guide the lay public. The 1968 Medicines Act brought in new rules about the licensing and labelling of herbal products and subsequent European legislation has continued to tighten these controls.

Under the 1968 rules all herbal medicines then available were subjected to a thorough review of their contents and efficacy. However, as an interim measure, existing lines were given until May 1990 to comply and

in the meantime were granted product licences as a right. They bore a code starting "PLR", which can still be seen on some anthroposophical products which have yet to undergo a full review.

New products introduced after 1968 had from the start to prove safety and efficacy before they hit the shelves. Under the Act medicines are defined as prescription only, pharmacy only and over-the-counter, and all preparations used as medicines and bearing a medicinal claim must be licensed.

Herbal remedies are strictly defined under the Act as "medicinal products consisting of a substance produced by subjecting a plant or plants to drying, crushing or any other process" – or a combination of such substances and water. Exemptions allow herbalists to make and supply herbal products to their patients without a licence and also exclude dried and crushed herbal products from the licensing rules – provided that the manufacturer gives no written recommendation on the package or in any accompanying leaflets about what that product might be used for. This exemption does not apply to imported products.

It means, however, that "echinacea capsules" or "marshmallow and peppermint tablets" do not need a licence and, strictly speaking, are not medicines at all. It also means that their packaging cannot explain that echinacea is a potent anti-bacterial ideal for infections or that marshmallow and peppermint pills can soothe gastritis and indigestion.

This can make buying unlicensed over-the-counter products very confusing as virtually no information about use can be found on many labels. One herbal supplier, for example, sells unlicensed remedies for arthritis as "Arthur's formula", while the anti-depressant

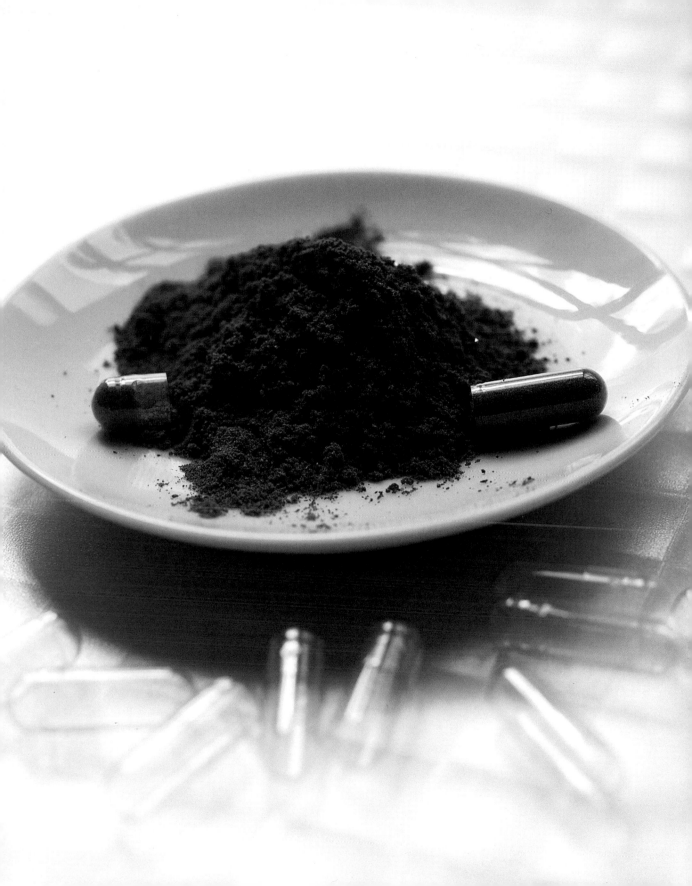

effects of St John's wort can only be hinted at in descriptions of the "sunshine herb".

Following the 1990 review of herbal products many traditional remedies that could not prove their effectiveness disappeared from the shelves. Those that were granted licences by the Medicines Control Agency have the product licence details (a code number starting PL) printed on the packages and can make carefully worded claims which generally start: "A herbal remedy traditionally used for the symptomatic relief of…". Such products usually also need to include an instruction to "consult your doctor if symptoms persist" on the label.

Because licences are only ever given for remedies used to treat minor self-limiting ailments, the printed claim is only a part of the picture. Products are not allowed to make claims for treating chronic problems, like arthritis or high blood pressure, so remedies that can tackle these ailments either have to be sold as suitable for something else or relegated to the unlicensed "food supplement" category.

Around a third of over-the-counter herbal products are actually licensed and a great many single herb remedies are, legally, sold as unlicensed supplements. Currently there are no licensed Ayurvedic and Chinese herbal preparations in Britain, and in some countries there are already bans on the importation of certain Chinese herbs, although as yet the UK remains reasonably liberal in its approach. Similarly, many herbal products licensed in other European countries have not been subject to the same rigorous review that the UK undertook back in 1990.

Similar sorts of legislation exist in other parts of the world. In Australia control is especially tight, with all herbal remedies needing to be licensed and stringent import controls restricting the use of many non-native plants. Numerous Chinese herbs, for example, cannot be imported and a wide range of fairly innocuous European herbs (such as periwinkle and borage) are also banned. In contrast, New Zealand has very minimal controls – rather like pre-1968 Britain – and many therapeutic claims are made, quite legally, for unlicensed products. This situation is likely to change in the future and a more controlled environment, as exists in Australia, is probable.

In the USA, control of herbal remedies has varied between states with some effectively banning almost all alternative therapies while others allow the over-the-counter sale of herbs that are more strictly regulated in other countries.

The over-the-counter market remains something of a minefield for the unwary. Always try to check actions in a herbal before buying to ensure that the product is going to be suitable, and be highly suspicious of products listing exotic ingredients or with dubious botanical names.

the **home** medicine **chest**

No one wants to fill the entire bathroom cabinet with herbal remedies, but keeping a limited selection at home to cope with minor ailments and first-aid problems is good sense. Ideal ingredients of the home herbal medicine chest would include:

Arnica – effective in improving circulation and encouraging healing, arnica creams can be used on chilblains, bruises and sprains. The herb should not be applied to broken skin as it is an irritant. Internally, homoeopathic doses (Arnica 6X or 30X) encourage recovery from surgery or traumatic injury.

Chickweed cream - made from the common garden weed – is often used to relieve the irritation of eczema, but it is also useful to soothe minor burns, sunburn and insect stings and can be helpful for drawing splinters and boils.

Cloves - essential oil of cloves is an ideal emergency standby for toothache (apply on a cotton wool swab) or insect bites. The tincture can be used instead of oil and also makes a warming remedy for stomach chills and nausea – use 10 drops of tincture in water.

Comfrey – this herb speeds up tissue growth and repair, so is good for bruises, sprains and even for healing fractures and cracked small bones. It can also be used on clean cuts. Use ointment or infused oil (see page 142-144 for cautions).

Echinacea tablets help combat colds, flu and infections. Always keep the first aid box well stocked with them.

Evening primrose or borage oil capsules can be helpful as an emergency hangover remedy to help restore normal liver function. Take 2-3 g on "the morning after" and try not to do it again! The oil can also be used neat on skin rashes.

Garlic tablets are useful for catarrh, coughs, to boost the immune system and to help reduce cholesterol levels. Low doses taken regularly can also help improve digestion function in the elderly.

Lavender oil, diluted in a vegetable-oil base, makes a helpful massage for headaches and muscular aches. It can also be used on insect bites and on minor burns and sunburn.

Passion flower tablets make a helpful sedative for anxiety and insomnia.

Slippery elm bark is an extremely mucilaginous herb largely used to soothe and protect against stomach inflammations. The powder can be made into a paste with a little water and taken for heartburn, gastritis, indigestion and for irritant coughs. It can also be used as a poultice or in ointments to draw splinters and corns. Tablets and capsules are a convenient alternative for internal use.

Tea tree oil is extracted from an Australian tree and is now known to be one of the most antiseptic and anti-fungal herbs available to us. The oil can be used neat on infected cuts or fungal infections, such as athlete's foot, while three or four drops on a tampon inserted in the vagina for up to three hours will help combat vaginal thrush. Creams are commercially available as an alternative.

Thyme and liquorice syrup is helpful for coughs and chest infections.

Distilled witch hazel is highly astringent, anti-inflammatory and stops bleeding. It can be used as a cooling lotion for minor burns, sunburn, bruises, insect bites and varicose veins, as well as on cuts, grazes and piles.

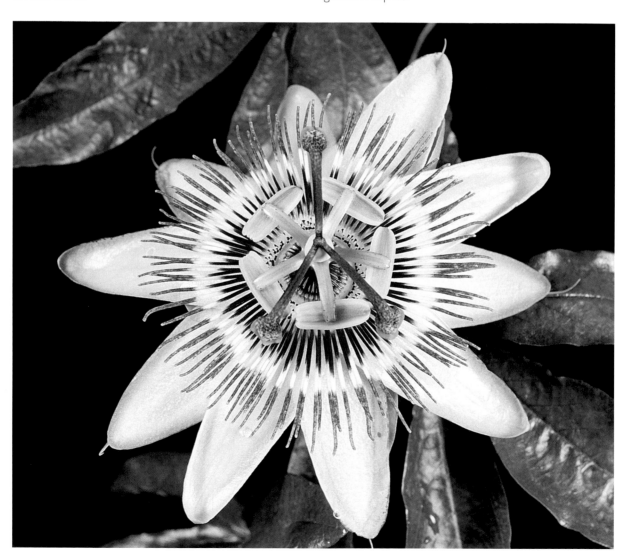

Passionflower *Passiflora incarnata*

Part 2: **all** sorts **of** remedies

We tend to think of herbs as some sort of "different" category of plants: something to relegate to a dedicated corner of the garden or to buy, dusty and faded, in a specialist shop. Healing plants are not always dreary "green things". They can come in all shapes and sizes from the humble vegetable to an exotic eastern flower. Many have their place in the home medicine chest and give plenty of choice for emergency first aid. This section provides information on some plants we would normally label as "herbs", but also on a number that we would more commonly find in the greengrocer's and others that can be discovered in field and woodland.

topically – anti-pruritic and anti-inflammatory; seeds – important source of essential fatty acids

The old country saying "borage for courage" is a rather apt description of the plant since we now know that it will stimulate the adrenal glands to secrete adrenaline – the "flight or fight" hormone which we produce in moments of stress. Borage has also long been regarded as uplifting for the emotions. It has been identified with the Roman *euphrosynum*, "the plant that cheers", which Pliny tells us was once added to wine to "increase the exhilarating effect", while Elizabethan cooks added blue borage flowers to salads to "make the mind glad". The herb is also soothing for irritant tissues, mildly sedative and anti-depressant. Externally the juice can be used to sooth itching skin.

In recent years borage has come to the fore as a rich source of *gamma*-linolenic acid (GLA) found in the pressed seed oil. Like evening primrose oil (see page 64), borage has thus become a favourite with the health food industry. GLA is one of the essential fatty acids needed by the body for a number of metabolic processes. Lack of it can be associated with menstrual irregularities, skin problems, irritable bowel syndrome and rheumatoid arthritis.

Borage oil is often sold as "starflower oil" – this is not a traditional name, but one which probably appeals to the marketeers. It contains substantially more GLA than evening primrose oil, with around 24% (compared with a figure of 9% generally quoted for evening primrose). However, traces of toxic erucic acid (which is known to damage heart tissue) are sometimes found in the oil, leading to claims that evening primrose oil is more efficacious.

Borage is also related to comfrey and traces of pyrrolizidine alkaloids – which can cause liver damage in large quantities – have been found in its leaves. It has therefore been banned in some countries, although most herbalists regard it as perfectly safe for regular use. The leaves can be used in teas for stress or to counter the lingering effects of steroid therapy and they can also be added to cough mixtures as an expectorant. The juice is available commercially or can be made by pulping the fleshy leaves in a food processor.

Marigold *Calendula officinalis*

Part used: flowers

Actions: astringent, antiseptic, anti-fungal, anti-inflammatory, antispasmodic, bile stimulant, bitter, diaphoretic, immune-stimulant, menstrual regulator, wound herb

Traditional English pot marigolds have been among the herbalist's favourites for centuries. In the 12th century simply looking at the plant's golden colour was supposed to lift the spirits and encourage cheerfulness – or as *Macer's Herbal* has it to "drawyth owt of ye heed wikked hirores [humours]". By Culpeper's day in the 17th century, marigold was recommended to "strengthen the heart" and was highly regarded as a remedy for smallpox and measles.

Today, marigold – often sold under its Latin name of calendula – is widely available in creams and ointments for cuts, grazes, fungal infections (including athlete's foot and vaginal thrush) and also for minor burns and skin disorders including dry eczema. Internally it is a useful

Marigold *Calendula officinalis*

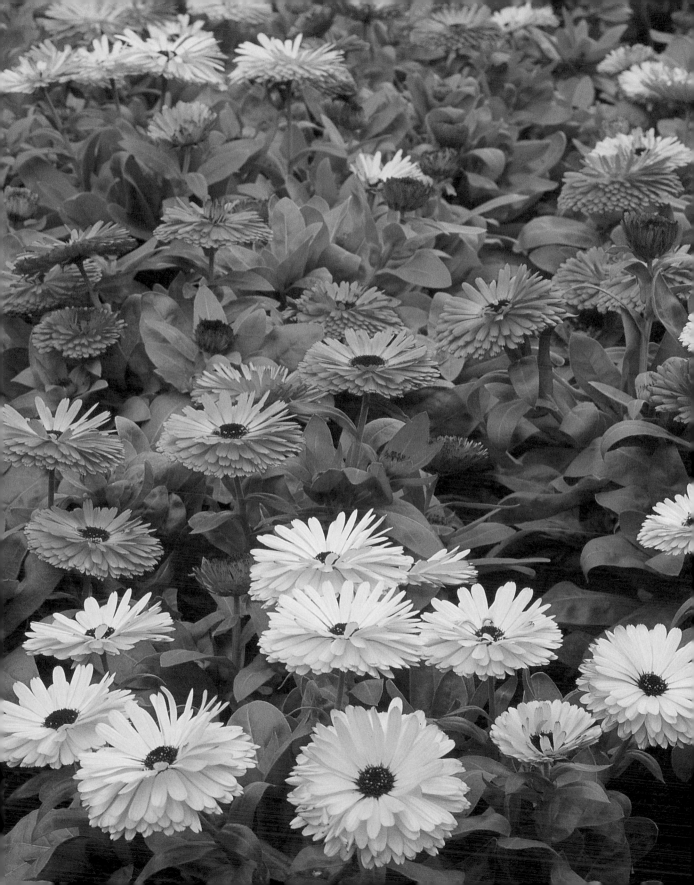

bitter to stimulate bile production and improve the digestion. It is ideal for a number of gynaecological problems, including irregular or painful menstruation, and it can also be used for gastric and gall bladder inflammations and as a cleansing remedy for inflamed lymph glands.

An infused oil can easily be made at home using the fresh or dried flowers (see pages 32-34), and this makes a good alternative to proprietary ointments. It can also be used as a base for essential oils (a few drops of tea tree, for example, can be added to make a strongly anti-fungal lotion for athlete's foot). The infused oil can be used to moisturise dry skin, added to bath water to ease eczema, or used as an antiseptic lotion for minor cuts and grazes.

The cream is also helpful for soothing sore nipples in breast feeding – an old-fashioned remedy which many maternity wards have now revived.

Echinacea *Echinacea* spp.

Parts used: root, aerial parts
Actions: antibiotic, anti-allergenic, anti-inflammatory, immune-stimulant, lymphatic tonic, vulnerary

Echinacea, or purple cone flower, was one of the most important herbs used by Native American healers. According to one 19th-century source it was used as a "remedy for more ailments than any other plant". The herb was treated as a universal antidote to snake bite, the juice was used to bathe burns and pieces of root were chewed for toothache.

By the 1850s echinacea was already widely used by European settlers, largely as an aromatic and carminative for digestive problems. Interest in the plant spread and by the 1930s research in Germany had highlighted its potent antibiotic actions.

The plant is anti-bacterial, anti-viral and anti-fungal and is used for a broad spectrum of infections. Today it is widely cultivated and regarded as one of the most useful herbs in the repertoire.

The roots of various related species are generally used medicinally, although preferences vary across Europe: the Germans favour the root of *E. pallida* while researchers there suggest that the aerial parts of *E. purpurea* are more efficacious than its root. In the UK we tend to use only the roots of both *E. purpurea* and *E. angustifolia* with *E. pallida* rarely found (partly because it can be harder to cultivate commercially). Harvesting aerial parts of home-grown specimens makes the herb a more practical alternative in the herb garden.

Attitudes to dosage of echinacea also vary, with some authorities suggesting that it should be taken in short sharp bursts of up to four weeks, while others happily feed low dosages to school-age children on a long-term basis, successfully preventing the usual round of childhood ills.

For general use, it is best to take echinacea in high doses at the first sign of a cold, using 10 ml of a 1:5 tincture or 3 x 200 mg capsules, three times daily for up to four days. For prophylactic use, exponents generally suggest one or two 200 mg capsules daily.

As well as treating colds, kidney and urinary infections, echinacea can also be used for wound healing and septicaemia. It is often sold as a licensed remedy for "minor skin problems", although it is really more suited to those associated with infection, such as acne, boils and carbuncles, rather than disorders like eczema which may have a more complex aetiology.

Siberian ginseng *Eleutherococcus senticosus*
Part used: root
Actions: adrenal stimulant, anti-viral, adaptagen, aphrodisiac, combats the actions of stress, immune-stimulant, lowers blood sugar levels, peripheral vasodilator, tonic

Despite its age – it belongs to one of the oldest known plant families, the Araliacaea – Siberian ginseng is a comparative newcomer to the West, "rediscovered" in the 1930s in Russia and subsequently extensively used by Soviet athletes to increase stamina and enhance performance.

It has been used in Chinese medicine for around 2,000 years and was traditionally regarded as a warming herb to strengthen the sinews and bones and to improve energy and blood flows, especially in the elderly. Its Chinese name, *Wu Jia Pi*, means "bark of five additions" – reminding us that the Chinese used only the root bark, not the whole root as in the West.

Siberian ginseng has been extensively researched and is known to stimulate the immune and circulatory systems and also help regulate blood pressure and lower blood sugar levels. As the Soviet researchers discovered back in the 1930s, it is also good at increasing stamina and helping the body cope more efficiently with both physical and mental stresses. It is ideal to take, normally as a tincture or in capsules, whenever extra energy is needed – before a particularly busy period at work, during exams or before long-distance air travel, for example. It can help reduce the effects of jet lag and is an ideal all-round energy tonic, considered to be rather gentler than Korean ginseng (see Ginseng, page 66) and more suitable for women.

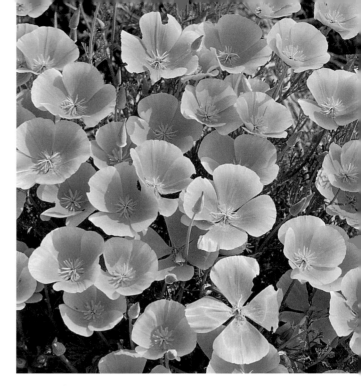

Californian poppy *Eschscholzia californica*

Californian poppy *Eschscholzia californica*
Parts used: aerial parts
Action: anodyne, diaphoretic, mild diuretic, sedative, relaxing nervine

Californian poppies are a popular and easy-to-grow garden plant with cheerful bright yellow flowers. Although a member of the poppy family, Californian poppy contains none of the alkaloids which depress the nervous system that its more potent relatives do. It is a mild soporific, suitable even for sleepless children. It has also been used to relieve pain.

For home use it is easy to gather the whole herb during the flowering season, dry in small bunches and store for use as a night-time tea to combat insomnia. Infuse two teaspoons of dried herb to one cup of boiling water for adults or half a teaspoon of dried herb for children. Sweeten with honey if required.

Eucalyptus *Eucalyptus globulus*

Parts used: leaves, essential oil

Actions: antiseptic, anti-spasmodic, anthelmintic, expectorant, febrifuge, lowers blood sugar levels, stimulant

The majority of eucalyptus species originate from Australia where the plant was widely used in Aboriginal medicine to treat fevers, dysentery and sores. In the 19th century, Baron Ferdinand von Müller, director of the Melbourne Botanical Gardens from 1857 to 1873, brought the plant to Europe and cultivation spread in southern Europe and North America. The tree is a greedy drinker and widespread cultivation in parts of Italy has since had a dramatic and adverse effect on local water-table levels.

The essential oil (extracted by steam distillation) is mainly used externally and is included in numerous rubs for muscle aches, steam inhalations for catarrh and colds, or added in small quantities to throat pastilles.

Various species are used medicinally, some of them with slightly different actions: Australian peppermint (*E. dives*) is largely used for chest rubs, sciatica and arthritis; lemon-scented eucalyptus (*E. citriodora*) has a more anti-fungal action and is used for athlete's foot and candidiasis. Russian research has suggested that some species are effective against the flu virus, others are anti-malarial or combat a wide range of bacteria.

Caution: Excess may cause headache and delirium.

Fennel *Foeniculum officinalis*

Parts used: seeds; the stem base is eaten as a vegetable

Actions: anti-inflammatory, carminative, circulatory stimulant, diuretic, mild expectorant, promotes the secretion of milk

Fennel has been cultivated since Roman times – grown for its thick bulbous stems which are used as a vegetable, while the feathery leaves are used in flavouring and the seeds in medicine. The Greeks called the plant *marathron,* which is reputedly derived from a verb meaning "to grow thin" and it seems to have been considered as an early slimming aid. Galen classified it as hot and dry, while later authors recommended it to counterbalance the cool, dampness of fish, or as Culpeper put it "…to consume the phlegmatic humour which fish most plentifully afford and annoy the body with".

Fennel was also associated with fortune telling and was used to decorate houses at midsummer to keep evil spirits at bay.

Today it is often used for indigestion, wind or colic and is added to laxative mixtures to ease the griping pains that strong purgatives can cause. Fennel tea bags are readily available and make a good after-dinner drink to ease the digestion. Fennel is also a good mouthwash for gum disease and sore throats and is sometimes included in herbal toothpastes. It is an ingredient in baby's gripe water – although an alternative in breast feeding is for the mother to drink fennel infusion so that baby receives its medicinal herbs with the daily milk.

The essential oil is sold commercially and can be added to external rubs for bronchial congestion.

Ginkgo *Ginkgo biloba*

Parts used: leaves, seeds

Actions: leaves – circulatory stimulant, vasodilator; seeds – anti-bacterial, anti-fungal, astringent

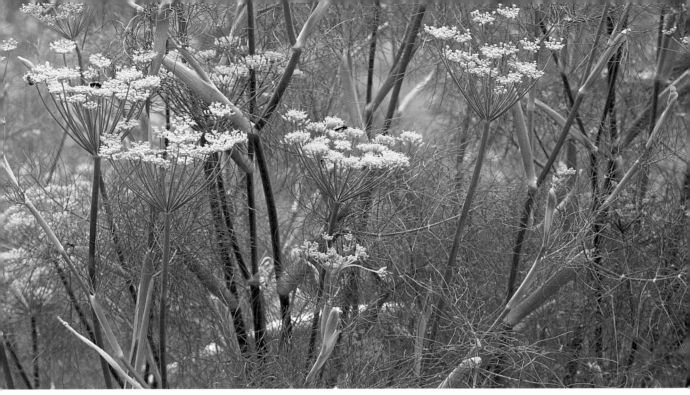

Fennel *Foeniculum officinalis*

Ginkgo is something of a botanical anachronism – a rare, prehistoric deciduous conifer, unchanged since before the evolution of mammals. It owes its survival to preservation as a sacred plant in Japanese temple gardens and was introduced into Europe in 1727 when it became popular as a botanical garden ornamental. Some of Europe's oldest ginkgo trees – also known as maidenhair trees – can be found in the Chelsea Physic Garden in London and the Jardin des Plantes in Paris.

Although the Chinese have prescribed the seeds for asthma and urinary problems for many centuries, it is only in the past few years that the herb has been used medicinally in the West. Research in the past decade has highlighted its action as a platelet-activating factor (PAF) which counters the allergic response – reinforcing its traditional use as an anti-asthmatic. More significantly, ginkgo has been shown to improve cerebral circulation. In Germany it has been tested on patients after brain surgery following strokes, and been found to improve recovery rates dramatically. Its action in strengthening the cerebral circulation has led many to regard it as an anti-ageing remedy, since hardening of the arteries in the brain is a common cause of apparent confusion in the elderly. It is generally beneficial for many circulatory ailments (including, according to some researchers, varicose veins) and its effect on cerebral circulation has also led to its use in the treatment of Ménières disease and tinnitus.

Ginkgo is widely sold as a food supplement and can be usefully taken by the elderly or those with chronic circulatory disorders. Typical dose is around 200 mg of extract or 2 g of powdered herb a day.

Liquorice *Glycyrrhiza glabra*

Part used: root

Actions: anti-arthritic, anti-inflammatory, antispasmodic, cooling, lowers cholesterol levels, expectorant, mild laxative, soothing for gastric mucosa, tonic stimulant for adrenal cortex, possibly anti-allergenic

Liquorice is one of our most widely researched and respected medicinal herbs: it has been used since at least 500 BC and drugs based on liquorice extracts are still listed in official pharmacopoeia as remedies for gastric ulcers and inflammation.

The Greeks called liquorice Sythian root and used it for asthma and coughs, while in traditional Chinese herbalism it is called the "great detoxifier" or "great harmoniser" and is believed to drive toxins and poisons from the system and also eliminate harmful side effects of other herbs.

The variety of liquorice used in Western herbal traditions is *G. glabra*: it originates in the Mediterranean region and Middle East and has been cultivated in Europe since at least the 16th century. The Chinese use an Asian species, *G. uralensis* (*Gan Cao*), which has similar actions. It is regarded as one of the most important of Chinese tonics – often called "the grandfather of herbs" – and pieces of Chinese liquorice root are often given to children to chew in order to promote muscle growth.

Liquorice has a hormonal effect, stimulating the adrenal cortex due to the presence of glycyrrhizin, which is some 50 times sweeter than sucrose, and encourages production of such hormones as hydrocortisone.

The plant is very soothing and demulcent, making it ideal for gastric ulceration. It is also a digestive stimulant and laxative and is often used for constipation.

Caution: Excessive liquorice can cause fluid retention and increase blood pressure and it should therefore be avoided by anyone suffering from hypertension. It should not be taken by those on digoxin-based drugs.

Witch hazel *Hamamelis virginiana*
Part used: bark
Actions: astringent, anti-inflammatory, styptic

The witch hazel tree was used for numerous ills by several Native American tribes: the Menomees in Wisconsin rubbed decoctions on their legs during sports to keep the muscles supple, while a maceration of the twigs was recommended for back ache. The Potawatomis preferred the twigs in steam baths for sore muscles, while a Dr Colden, writing to a colleague in Leyden in 1744, describes how the Mohawks used steam from witch hazel decoctions to treat eye injuries and records a case of "almost total blindness occasioned by a blow" cured by this method.

The plant has been growing in Europe since the 17th century and its botanical name derives from a Greek word suggesting a resemblance to the apple tree. It is a small, shrub-like tree growing to around 5 m in height and with yellow flowers in spring.

The bark is steam distilled to produce the familiar, clear "distilled witch hazel" available from any pharmacy. It can be used as a first-aid remedy for bruises, sprains, nosebleeds, cuts and grazes, can soothe spots and blemishes, and is helpful to ease varicose veins and piles. It is ideal for all sorts of minor household injuries. The tincture of the bark, well diluted, can be used much as commercially made generic distilled witch hazel; a number of proprietary creams and ointments are available.

Taken internally, an infusion of the leaves is effective for treating diarrhoea, colitis, excessive menstruation and haemorrhage.

Devil's claw *Harpagophytum procumbens*
Part used: root
Actions: anti-inflammatory, anti-rheumatic, mild analgesic, bile stimulant, cleansing, reputed cortisone-like activity, diuretic, lymphatic stimulant, sedative

Devil's claw has been known in the West for less than 100 years, although the plant has long been used in folk medicine by the Bushmen of the Kalahari Desert in southern Africa, where it grows wild. The herb takes its name from its large thorny seed pods which are a hazard for animals when they become entangled in fur – its botanical name is derived from the Greek *harpago*, meaning a grappling hook.

The story of devil's claw's discovery by Western medicine exists in several versions: the plant was variously spotted by a Boer farmer or German doctor, being variously used by local people or a tribal witch doctor to cure digestive upsets or rheumatism, and was subsequently despatched to Germany for investigation. Certainly by the late 1950s its anti-inflammatory and anti-rheumatic properties were well established. Researchers found that constant use of the herb for at least six weeks significantly improved the movement of arthritic joints and reduced swelling.

Some 40 constituents have been identified although, as their action is not well understood, the whole plant extract is always used: it is generally sold in over-the-counter products as a "simple" – singly in capsules or tinctures rather than in combination with other herbs. Devil's claw is bitter and can be used as a digestive stimulant. Externally it can be used in creams and rubs for muscle and joint pains. The herb has become a popular over-the-counter product and is widely available.

Caution: Devil's claw is believed to stimulate uterine contractions and should be avoided in pregnancy.

Hops *Humulus lupulus*
Part used: strobiles (flowers from female plants)
Action: anaphrodisiac, bitter digestive stimulant, diuretic, sedative, restoring tonic for nervous system

Although we associate hops with traditional English beer, the plant is a comparative newcomer, introduced from Germany in the 16th century. Enthusing about the hop's many virtues, John Gerard, writing in 1597, urges that "beer" be considered a "phisicall drink to keep the body in health [rather] than an ordinary drinke for the quenching of our thirst", while a few years earlier (1562) William Turner in his *New Herball* was amazed that, given the herb's numerous properties, physicians did not "use it more in medicine".

Just as in brewing, the female flowers or strobiles are used medicinally. They are strongly sedating, so should be avoided by those liable to depression. Their anaphrodisiac action may be familiar to beer drinkers: excessive consumption can lead to loss of libido. This action is due to oestrogen-like compounds in the plant: women hop pickers often experienced menstrual irregularities and early periods while working in the hop fields and breathing in the herb's potent aromatic oils.

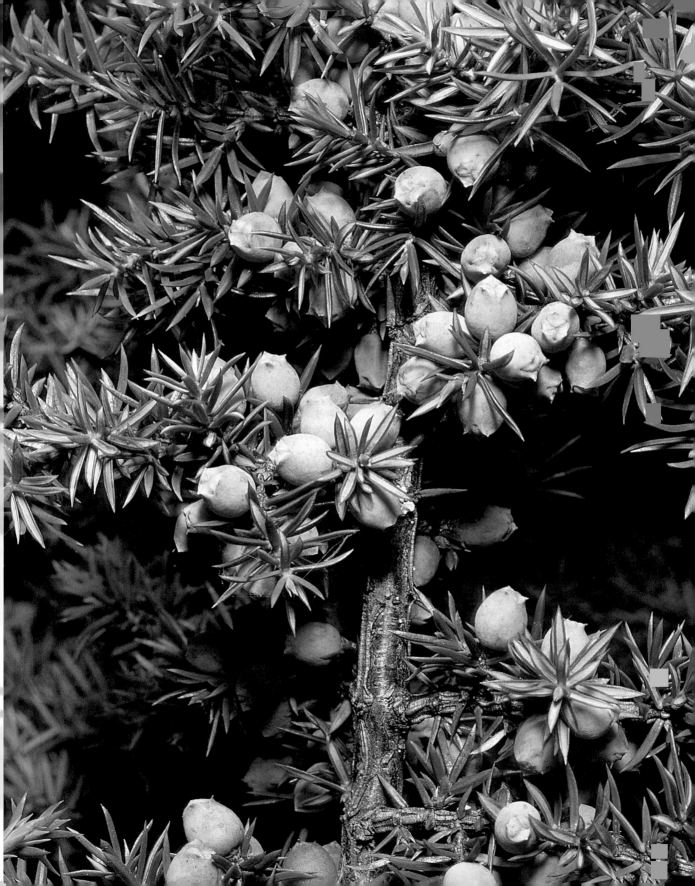

1550 BC. A type of juniper (*J. phoenica*) was grown in Egypt and tomb paintings showing the berries being picked and processed survive in the Saqqara tombs built around 2300 BC.

Juniper berries are widely used for urinary tract problems, such as cystitis, and as a cleansing remedy for rheumatism. The essential oil, collected by steam-distilling the berries, is used in aromatherapy both for urinary problems and as a stimulating tonic massage. The same oil is added as a flavouring to London gin – hence the diuretic action of that particular beverage. Another type of oil made from juniper is cade oil, produced by dry-distilling the heartwood of various juniper species and used for psoriasis and other skin problems It contains phenol and is mildly disinfectant.

Caution: Prolonged use of juniper can irritate the kidneys and any preparation containing the herb should not be taken for longer than six weeks without professional advice. It should not be taken internally by those suffering from kidney disease and high doses must be avoided in pregnancy.

Lavender *Lavandula angustifolia*
Parts used: flowers, essential oil
Actions: analgesic, anti-bacterial, anti-depressant, anti-spasmodic, carminative, bile stimulant, circulatory stimulant, relaxant, tonic for the nervous system

The name lavender comes from the Latin *lavare*, to wash, and the herb has been used to scent baths and toiletries since Roman times. Lavender is useful for

Juniper *Juniperus communis*

digestive upsets, nervous tension, insomnia, migraines and headaches. The flowers can be made into a pleasant tasting tea taken at night for sleeplessness or during the day for headaches and nervous tension.

Dioscorides, writing in the second century AD, recommended lavender for "griefs in the thorax", although the plant used by the Greeks was probably *L. stoechas*, generally known today as French lavender and rather less hardy than the familiar English variety. In Arabic medicine this tradition of using lavender for chest problems has continued and it is still used in the Middle East as an expectorant.

Herbalists usually describe lavender as "cooling", suggesting that it is best suited to ease those sorts of headaches that are soothed by cold packs rather than the sort of pain that is comforted by a warm compress.

The essential oil is steam-distilled from the flowers and is used in aromatherapy for muscular aches, pains and headaches (add 1 ml lavender oil to 20 ml of sunflower oil and massage into painful areas). A few drops of lavender oil can also be added to creams for eczema or diluted in water to make a soothing lotion for sunburn and minor scalds. Added to bath water, lavender oil is relaxing and soothing for nervous tensions and insomnia; in massage oils it can be helpful for muscular aches and pains, strains and some rheumatic problems.

Chamomile *Matricaria recutita/Chamaemelum nobile*
Part used: flowers
Actions: anti-emetic, anti-inflammatory, antispasmodic, bitter, carminative, sedative

Both German chamomile (*M. recutita*) and its relative Roman chamomile (*C. nobile*) are among the most

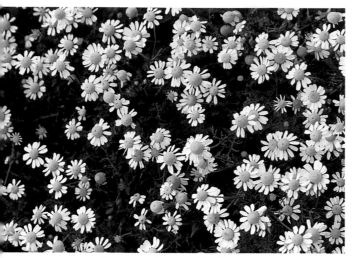

German chamomile *Matricaria recutita*

widely used of medicinal herbs. Their actions are very similar, with Roman chamomile having a slightly more bitter taste and German chamomile being slightly more anti-inflammatory and analgesic. While herbalists may have their individual favourites the plants are extremely close in action and can be regarded as interchangeable in lay use.

The Greeks knew the herb as "ground apple" (*kamai melon*) — so called because of its characteristic smell — and it is still used for ornamental lawns, giving a hint of apples when walked on. Special non-flowering cultivars have been developed for lawns, but these are useless if you want to use the herb medicinally since it is only the flowers that are of value.

To the Anglo-Saxons chamomile was *maythen*, one of the nine sacred herbs given to mankind by Woden and listed in the ninth-century poem the *Lacnunga*.

Both chamomiles are used for nervous stomach upsets, nausea, insomnia, and externally in creams for eczema, wounds, nappy rash, sore nipples and piles. The flowers are readily available in tea bags or sold loose for

infusions and, although the flavour can be something of an acquired taste, chamomile tea is probably one of the most popular herbal drinks on the market.

Chamomile is also used in homoeopathy and Chamomilla 3X is a valuable standby for babies, used to treat both colic and teething. It is one of the safest herbs for children and babies and some mothers use weak infusions as a night-time drink to encourage restful sleep. The infusion can also be added to bath water to soothe over-excited infants.

Chamomile yields a deep blue essential oil on steam distillation which is very relaxing and useful in skin care. This is used for a range of digestive disorders, inflammations, emotional problems and muscle pains. It is extremely expensive but usually 2-3 drops are sufficient.

The botanists have renamed chamomile repeatedly over the years — Roman chamomile may still be found labelled as *Anthemis nobile* while German chamomile is often called either *Chamomilla recutita* or *Matricaria chamomilla*.

Tea tree *Melaleuca alternifolia*
Part used: essential oil
Actions: anti-bacterial, anti-fungal, antiseptic, anti-viral, diaphoretic, expectorant

Extracts from the Australian tea tree were originally used by the Aborigines as a wound remedy and by the Second World War it was a regular component in field dressing kits among Australian troops. The plant was first studied in Europe in the 1920s when French researchers found that tea tree oil, collected by steam distillation, was a more effective antiseptic than phenol and also identified its impressive antibiotic properties.

In the past few years a thriving tea tree industry has grown up which has led to a number of highly adulterated oils appearing on the market. True tea tree oil is one of the few which does not usually irritate mucous membranes and it can be used neat on the skin. A few drops added to tampons make a topical treatment of vaginal thrush (insert and leave them for no longer than four hours). Tea tree oil also stimulates the immune system and if taken internally (not recommended without professional guidance) acts as an expectorant and diaphoretic, making it useful for chills and coughs.

Tea tree is readily available both as oil and in creams and is an essential household standby for use in antiseptic dressings for cuts and grazes, for acne and other skin infections, or applied to all sorts of fungal infections (including thrush and athlete's foot).

A drop of tea tree oil can help prevent cold sores developing if applied as soon as the pricking sensation that heralds the sore starts, or it can help soothe them once they appear. It is also effective on warts, verrucas and insect bites. The oil, used neat on a comb or added to shampoos, can be used for head lice and nits in children.

Lemon balm *Melissa officinalis*

Parts used: aerial parts, essential oil
Actions: anti-bacterial, anti-depressant, anti-viral, diaphoretic, digestive stimulant, peripheral vasodilator, relaxing, restorative for the nervous system, sedative

Lemon balm's botanical name, *Melissa,* comes from the Greek word *mel*, meaning honey, and the herb has a long association with bees and the healing power of their products. It was regarded by the Greeks as a cure-all while the plant is said to be such a favourite with bees that if hives are rubbed with its leaves the insects will never swarm and always return. Lemon balm has been considered over the centuries as being as valuable as honey for treating wounds and equal in tonic effect to royal jelly.

John Gerard declared that it "comforteth the hart and driveth away all melancholie and sadnesse", while it was praised by Paracelsus as an "elixir of youth" which he made into a preparation called *primum ens melissae*. As late as the 18th century lemon balm was still being recommended in "canary wine" to "renew youth".

Today we regard the plant more prosaically as a carminative and sedative – useful to reduce body temperature in fever and a gentle herb for treating nervous tummy upsets in children. It is, however, potent enough to help with depression and anxiety and to relieve tension headaches.

Variegated lemon balm *Melissa officinalis aurea*

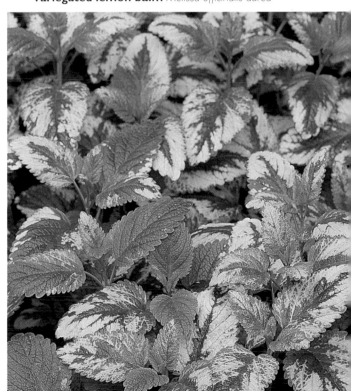

Tea made from a handful of fresh leaves makes a refreshing and restorative drink at the end of the day, although it needs to be dried with care to avoid losing too much of the characteristic lemon flavour. Externally, lemon balm creams can be used on insect bites, sores and slow-healing wounds. The essential oil is used in aromatherapy for nervous problems but is also valuable, well-diluted in sprays, for keeping insects away.

Peppermint *Mentha x piperita*

Part used: leaves

Actions: analgesic, anti-emetic, antispasmodic, carminative, bile stimulant, digestive tonic, peripheral vasodilator, diaphoretic but also cooling internally

There are thought to be around 30 different species of mint – but as the plants readily cross-pollinate and hybridise no-one is really certain. As the monk Wilafrid Strabo put it about 875 AD "…if a man can name the full list of all the kinds and all the properties of mint, he must know how many fish swim in the Indian Ocean".

Peppermint is the variety most widely used in herbal medicine, and is believed to be a cross between spearmint (*M. spicata*) and water mint (*M. aquatica*): it has a high menthol content – hence the characteristic smell. Until the 17th century there was little differentiation between the species – peppermint would just as often have been used in "mint sauce" as the apple mint (*M. suaveolens*) we favour today. Spearmint, also known as common mint or garden mint, is the variety most often grown in gardens and makes an adequate substitute for peppermint used medicinally. It does not have the high menthol content of peppermint, so is far less irritant and can be more suitable for children.

In general all the mints are antispasmodic, carminative, diaphoretic and decongestant. Peppermint oil is also antiseptic and mildly anaesthetic. Mints stimulate the digestion – drink a cup of peppermint or spearmint tea after meals – and are warming and decongestant in colds and catarrh. Peppermint, taken in tea, tincture or tablet form, can help to relieve nausea (including morning sickness), while the oil is used in stimulating rubs to soothe rheumatism and bronchial congestion.

Caution: Peppermint should not be given to babies or toddlers in any form: excess of the oil can irritate the stomach lining and misuse may lead to ulceration. The herb can also cause an allergic reaction in sensitive individuals.

Evening primrose *Oenothera biennis*

Part used: seed oil

Actions: alterative, hormone regulator, source of essential fatty acids

A native of North America, evening primrose is now widely naturalised across Europe and is commonly found in hedgerows as a garden escapee. The leaves were traditionally used for asthma and digestive disorders; however, during the 1970s researchers identified that the seeds are rich in an essential fatty acid called *gamma*-linolenic acid (GLA) that is vital for good health.

GLA is a building block for various prostaglandins – hormone-like chemicals vital for a number of bodily systems. A normal, healthy metabolism will convert commonly occurring *cis*-linoleic acid (found in leafy

Evening primrose *Oenothera biennis*

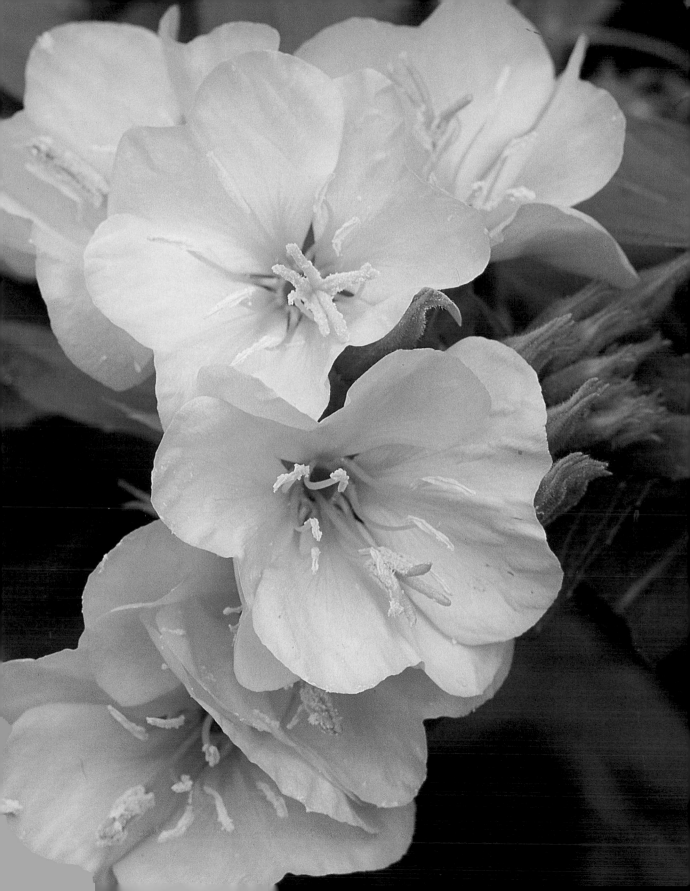

vegetables and seed oils) into GLA, but this process can be affected by poor diet and high cholesterol levels. Some individuals are also unable to complete this metabolic pathway – a failure that has been linked to disorders such as chronic psoriasis and rheumatoid arthritis. With evening primrose oil able to fill the gap, there has been a massive growth in sales and the plant has become a major cash crop in many parts of the world. Typically evening primrose oil contains around 9% GLA, although in recent years plant breeders have worked hard to develop strains that will yield even more.

GLA is also reputed to ease menstrual and menopausal problems, strengthen the circulatory system, combat certain sorts of eczema and boost the immune system. Research suggests that it can ease irritable bowel syndrome where symptoms are associated with the menstrual cycle. In clinical trials dosages of 3-5 g a day have been commonplace, although for general use most suppliers recommend 500-1000 mg. The oil can also be used neat on the skin for eczema and similar problems. Because the oil also helps to normalise liver function it can be useful to counter the symptoms of a hangover on "the morning after".

Licensed evening primrose oil products are available and, in the UK, can be prescribed for skin problems under the NHS. In the 1980s GLA was also found in borage (see page 49) and blackcurrant seed oils.

Ginseng *Panax ginseng*
Part used: root
Actions: aphrodisiac, reduces blood sugar and cholesterol levels, immune stimulant, stimulant, tonic

Ginseng has been regarded as something of a "wonder drug" for at least 5,000 years. Originating in China – where it has long been used to strengthen the vital energy, or *Qi*, of the body – the herb was known to Arab physicians by the ninth century, mentioned by Marco Polo in the 13th and introduced into modern Europe in the 17th century when a delegation from the King of Siam visited Louis XIV at Versailles and presented him with a root of "*gintz-æn*".

Ginseng has always been an expensive and highly prized herb that had, ideally, to be gathered in the wild using roots that were several years old. Today most ginseng is cultivated and it is an important cash crop. The plant is rich in steroidal compounds which are very similar to human sex hormones – hence its reputation as an aphrodisiac.

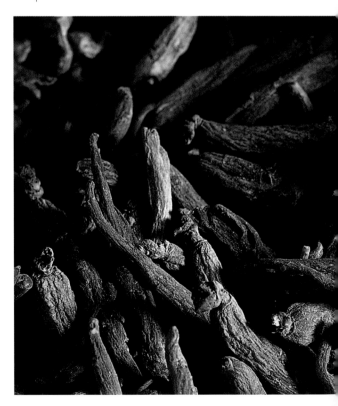

Ginseng *Panax ginseng*

The Chinese believe it is best suited to the elderly, preferring other energy tonics for those under 40, while many herbalists regard it as more suitable for men than women since it raises *yang* energy. The Chinese also believe it acts on the lungs and spleen and so can be helpful during recovery from chest problems – such as asthma – and digestive disorders.

As a general tonic it is ideally taken for a month in late autumn when the weather is changing from hot summer to cold winter and the body needs to adapt to the new environment, although the herb can, of course, be taken whenever there are problems due to tiredness and overwork.

A wide choice of over-the-counter products is available; typical dose is 600 mg of the root extract daily.

Cautions: Ginseng is best avoided in pregnancy although it may be taken then in small quantities for short periods. Other herbal stimulants, such as caffeine-containing drinks and horseradish – should be avoided while taking ginseng.

Passion flower *Passiflora incarnata*
Parts used: aerial parts
Action: analgesic, antispasmodic, bitter, cooling, hypotensive, sedative

Passion flower takes its name not from any effect it may have on the emotions, but from the religious symbolism of its flowers: the three stigmas were taken to represent the nails of the Crucifixion, the five anthers were Christ's five wounds, while the ten petals represented the Apostles present at the time (Peter and Judas Iscariot having absented themselves).

The herb is known as maypop in North America and was traditionally used by the Houmas in Louisiana as a blood tonic while the Mayans regarded the crushed plant as helpful for swellings and the decoction for ringworm. It was first described by a European botanist in the 1780s and by the 19th century had joined the herbal repertoire, initially as a remedy for epilepsy and later as a cure for insomnia.

Today, it is considered as an effective but gentle sedative and painkiller which will also reduce blood pressure. Passion flower is widely used in over-the-counter products for anxiety and nervous tension and is often combined with valerian or hops. An infusion of the dried herb can also be helpful for period pain or tension headaches, and can be supportive for a number of other nervous conditions such as irritable bowel syndrome and irregular heart beats.

Isphaghula *Plantago* spp.
Parts used: seeds, seed husks
Action: anti-bacterial, anti-diarrhoeal, anti-inflammatory, demulcent, bulking laxative

Popularly sold under a variety of brand names, the black psyllium or flea seeds (*P. psyllium*) and pinkish-brown isphaghula (*P. ovata*) are among the most popular of prescription and over-the-counter bulking laxatives. Both seeds and husks are available and both need to be soaked in water (1 teaspoon to a cup of boiling water) to produce a mucilaginous mixture which is then swallowed to encourage peristalsis and lubricate the bowel.

Many find this glutinous mixture rather hard to take, hence the large number of proprietary capsules which are simply swallowed with water so that the seeds

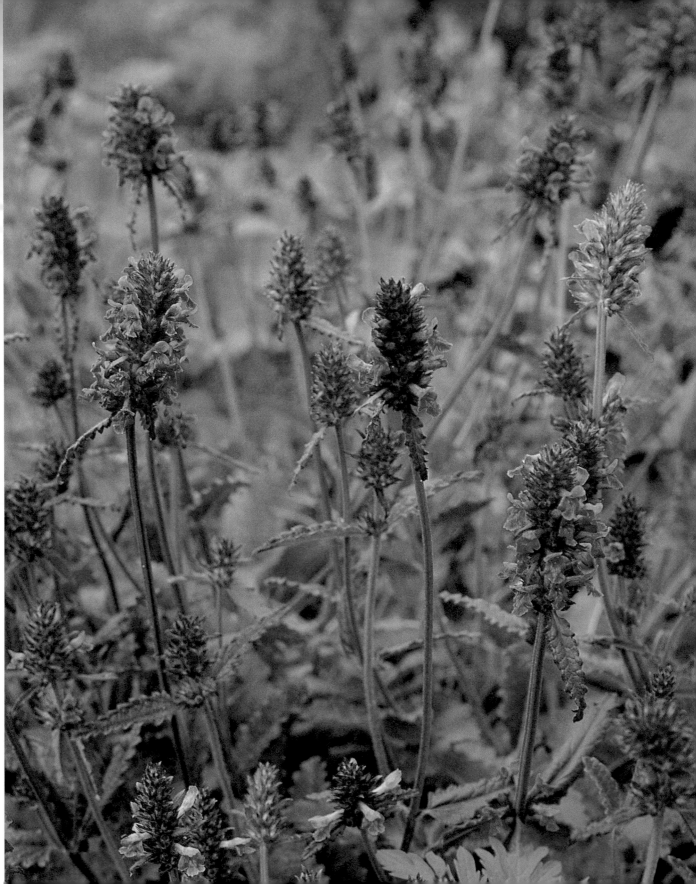

lactating mothers on weaning. The plant has an affinity with the throat and makes an excellent gargle and mouth wash for minor infections and inflammations.

The purple variety (*S. officinalis* Purpurascens Group) is often preferred by herbalists, although other cultivars display similar properties. Use in a tea for indigestion or drink a cup regularly as a tonic to combat the effects of old age. In many parts of Europe, sage ointment is a favourite standby for minor cuts and insect bites.

In China the roots of a related plant, *Salvia miltiorhiza*, known as *Dan Shen*, are used as a cooling sedative and energy tonic which will also stimulate blood flow.

Skullcap *Scutellaria lateriflora*
Parts used: aerial parts
Actions: anti-bacterial, antispasmodic, cooling, digestive stimulant, hypotensive, lowers cholesterol levels, relaxing and restorative nervine, styptic

Virginian skullcap was first introduced into Europe in the 18th century and was used as a treatment for rabies – hence its alternative name of "mad dog". It was used by the Cherokee to encourage menstruation and also to treat diarrhoea and breast pains. Today it is mainly considered as a sedative and nervine by Western herbalists but may also be used to reduce fevers, calm the foetus and stimulate the digestion.

Like all skullcaps, the plant takes its name from the dish-shaped seed pods, while its botanical name is derived from the growing pattern of the flowers which appear on only one side of the stem. Virginian skullcap grows easily in British gardens and will self-seed

Wood betony *Stachys officinalis*

enthusiastically – to the point where it can become invasive. European skullcap species (such as *S. galericulata*) have very similar properties although there is little tradition of using them in herbal medicine.

Drink skullcap tea to encourage relaxation and combat anxiety and nervous tension. Skullcap tea can also be useful to soothe pre-menstrual tension.

In China the root of *S. baicalensis* (*Huang Qin*) is regarded as a cooling remedy for the stomach and lungs and is used to clear "heat" which in Chinese theory may cause diarrhoea, jaundice and gastro-enteritis. This variety of skullcap is also anti-bacterial, antispasmodic, diuretic and will stimulate bile flow.

Wood betony *Stachys officinalis*
Parts used: aerial parts
Actions: astringent, bitter digestive remedy, circulatory tonic particularly for cerebral circulation, nervine, sedative

Although wood betony tends to be rather neglected these days, it was one of the most important healing plants in the Anglo-Saxon repertoire: no fewer than 29 uses of it are known and as well as recommending it for a range of physical diseases, it was a popular amulet herb used well into the Middle Ages – tied on to the arm with red wool – to ward off evil or ill humours. As late as 1526 *The Grete Herball* was recommending it "for them that be ferful", while William Turner, in 1551, advises that it will heal "them that are mad" and John Gerard (1597) gives a very long list of applications concluding that "it maketh a man to pisse well".

The herb is an attractive one for the garden with bright cerise flowers in late summer to autumn. It is mainly used these days as a nervine and sedative for headaches and nervous debility and makes a pleasant-tasting tea. It is also a good anti-catarrhal herb and, taken in a tea or tincture, can help reduce the discomfort of sinusitis and severe nasal congestion.

Culpeper, in 1653, stressed that it "preserves the liver and bodies of men from epidemical diseases and from witchcraft" and it certainly has an affinity with the liver – ideal for poor or sluggish digestion, and as a general stimulant. It can be especially helpful for menopausal problems.

Cautions: Although helpful during labour, wood betony should be avoided in pregnancy as it is a uterine stimulant.

Feverfew *Tanacetum parthenium*
Part used: leaves
Actions: anti-inflammatory, analgesic, antispasmodic, anthelmintic, cooling, digestive stimulant, emmenagogue, peripheral vasodilator, relaxant

Like comfrey, feverfew has hit the media headlines in recent years – this time as a major "cure" and prophylactic for migraine and arthritis. Since the 1970s, the plant has been extensively researched and is known to contain parthenolides and similar compounds which are believed to account for its action in easing the symptoms of both migraine and chronic arthritis. As an antispasmodic it can be helpful for period pain and is useful for minor fevers.

Although there is some tradition of using feverfew for headaches this was largely in external applications – writing in 1640, the herbalist John Parkinson suggested that the leaves were too bitter and unpleasant to eat: so in order to treat headaches, he recommended that they should be made into a poultice and placed on the crown of the head. Today, rightly or wrongly, they are one of the most popular over-the-counter herbs for treating migraines – although the bitter substances they contain do have a tendency to cause mouth ulcers in a significant number of users.

The name feverfew does not allude to some ancient major use as a febrifuge but is a corruption of feather-few – a description of its fine petals.

Clinical trials have well demonstrated its efficacy as a migraine remedy and many sufferers happily eat a couple of leaves a day as a prophylactic. The herb does, however, have anti-platelet activity, reducing the blood's ability to clot, so should not be taken by those on blood-thinning drugs.

Caution: Not to be taken by those prescribed warfarin, heparin and similar drugs. Migraine sufferers should stop taking regular doses of feverfew if side effects (skin rashes or mouth ulceration) occur.

Thyme *Thymus vulgaris*
Parts used: aerial parts, essential oil
Actions: antibiotic, antiseptic, antispasmodic, anti-microbial, anti-tussive, astringent, carminative, diuretic, expectorant, wound herb; topically rubefacient

Like many culinary herbs thyme is a soothing digestive remedy which can stimulate the digestion as it copes with rich foods. The plant (particularly the oil) is also

One of the many cultivars of thyme *Thymus spp.*

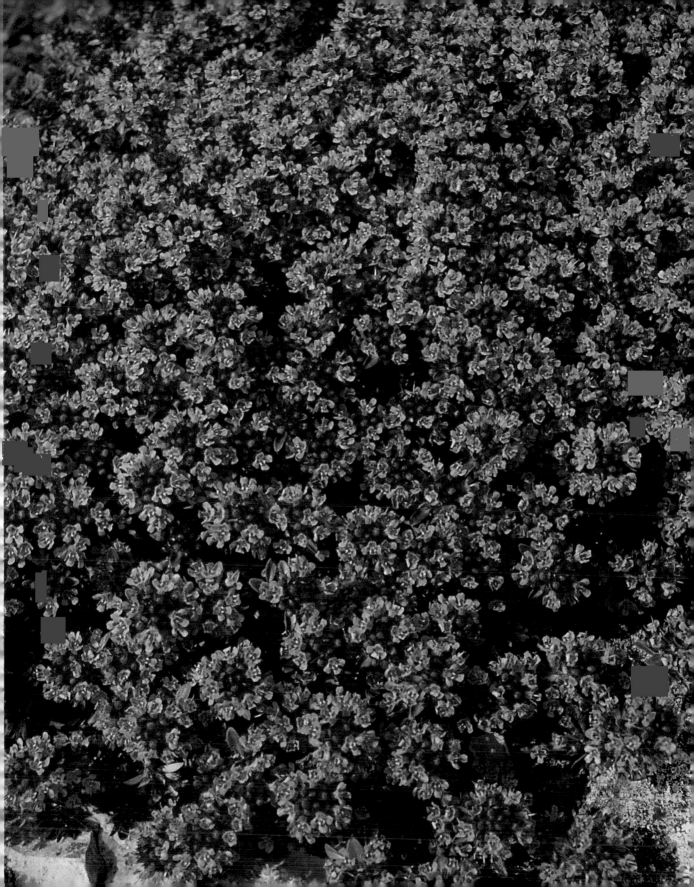

wives tales" of vervain that told of "witchcraft and sorceries". As late as the 17th century the plant was still being used in fortune-telling rites – a practice that can be traced back at least to Druidic times.

The Romans called it *hiera botane* (sacred plant) and used it to purify homes and spread on Jupiter's altars. Well into the Christian era it was castigated as a witch plant – or, as the 11th-century Physicians of Myddfai warned, "Give no heed to those who say that it should be gathered in the name of the devil." The Druids, according to Pliny, collected it when the "dog star could be seen in the heavens" and even today many regard it as a strong spiritual herb capable of healing holes in the human aura.

Medicinally it is largely used as a nervine and liver tonic – bitter and stimulating for the digestion – and an ideal tonic in convalescence and debility. It is sedating and is included in a number of over-the-counter remedies for anxiety and stress. It can also be helpful for neuralgia and migraine – taken internally or applied topically in the form of a compress. Vervain combines well with oats for combating depression and is a useful herb for nursing mothers – relaxing the nervous system to take the tension out of feeding time and stimulating milk flow.

Caution: Vervain should be avoided in pregnancy but can be taken in labour to stimulate contractions.

Chaste-tree *Vitex agnus-castus*
Part used: fruit
Actions: female aphrodisiac, male anaphrodisiac, pituitary stimulant, reproductive tonic

In recent years *Vitex agnus-castus* has become one of the most popular herbs for a range of gynaecological problems. It acts on the pituitary gland to increase the production of female sex hormones involved in ovulation, so can help to regulate the menstrual cycle and also improve hormone production at the menopause.

The herb is known as chaste-tree and grows wild in Mediterranean areas including Greece and Turkey, where it is regarded in folk medicine as a potent female aphrodisiac. Some argue that the common name is derived from its pure white flowers, although an equally likely explanation derives from its use as a male anaphrodisiac in medieval times. Then, the herb was taken by celibate monks to reduce libido and lascivious thoughts – hence its alternative country name of monk's pepper. It is still sometimes prescribed for problems with premature ejaculation.

For women, it is considered best to take chaste-tree in the early morning when the pituitary gland is believed to be most active. Low doses – 10-20 drops of a 1:5 tincture – are often preferred. In higher doses it sometimes has the side effect of "formication" – a sensation generally described as ants crawling over the skin.

Chaste tree *Vitex agnus-castus*

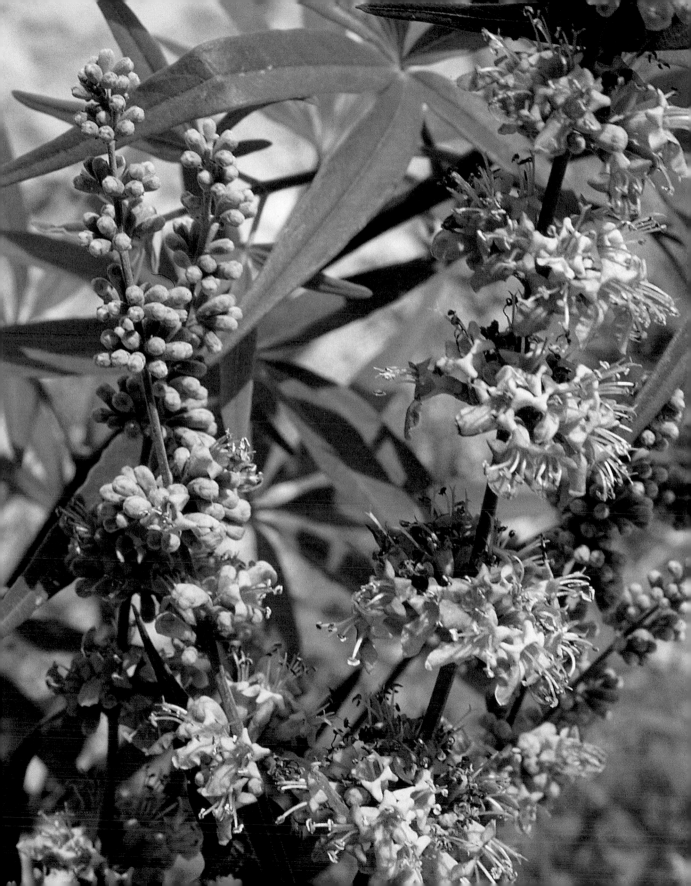

household healers

A very fine grey line divides the concept of "food" from that of "herbal medicine": many plants sit comfortably in both categories while herbal suppliers often prefer to describe their products as "food supplements" to avoid the need for complex medical licensing.

Many medicinal herbs − including some covered in the previous section − are valuable seasonings, while herbs that we think of primarily as cooking additives − such as dill (*Anethum graveolens*) or parsley − also have medicinal properties. The same applies to plants that we categorise as "foods". Onions, apples, cabbages, even cold tea all have their therapeutic properties and can be used as emergency remedies.

Equally, we need to remember the actions of these foods, as a surfeit can produce as many side effects as an overdose of a more orthodox "drug": how many of us have eaten rather too many peaches, nectarines or plums when the fruits arrive in the shop only to wonder at the sudden bout of diarrhoea that follows? All these fruits would be described by orthodox practitioners as "laxative", which explains the problem. To the 17th-century doctor, however, they would have been classified as "cold" and generally rather "moist" as well; the intrinsic coldness of the fruit would be blamed for any troublesome digestive problems that followed.

In Galenical medicine, foods were not only necessary nutrients, as we have seen (page 7), they each had particular characteristics that could affect the healthy balance of the system and so they had to be used in moderation or carefully combined to avoid side effects. These traditions still survived in Culpeper's day, although by then the practice was falling from use: "One good old fashion is not yet left off," he wrote in 1653, "viz. to boil fennel with fish: for it consumes that phlegmatic humour which fish most plentifully afford and annoy the body with, though few that use it know wherefore they do it."

While modern medicine dismisses humoral theories as medieval hocus pocus, scientists do at least acknowledge that sometimes foods are not always as safe as we would believe. Man-made hazards (such as BSE) apart, foods often contain toxic chemicals which can do harm as well as good and in excess they can sometimes seem to present as many troublesome side effects as more orthodox medicines.

For an explanation of any unfamiliar terms in the following pages, consult the glossary on pages 183-185; for advice on typical dosages and on preparing your own remedies, see pages 24-40.

Onions *Allium cepa*

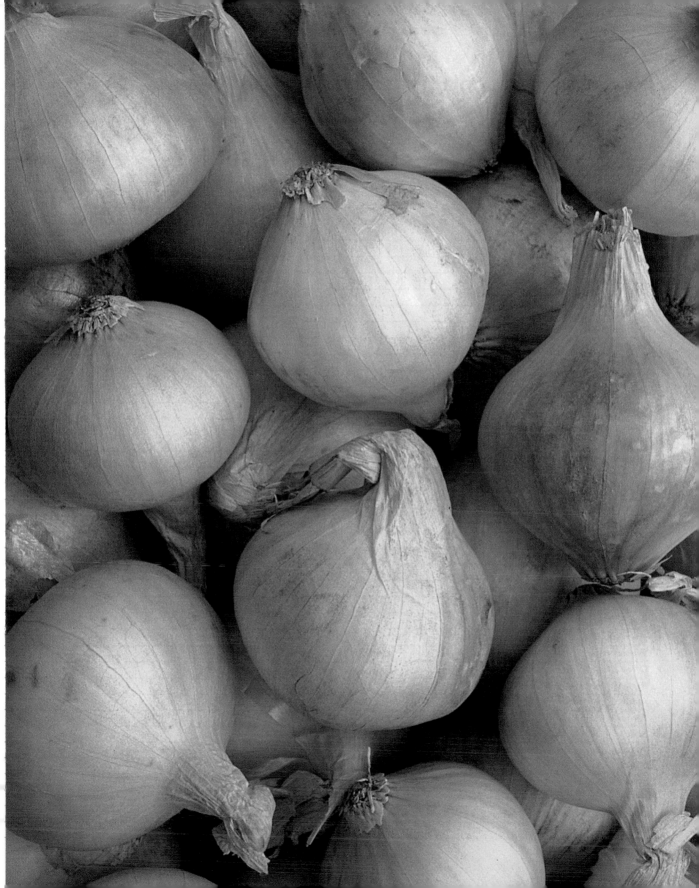

Asparagus *Asparagus officinalis*
Part used: stem
Actions: cleansing, diuretic, laxative, liver stimulant, reputed sedative for the heart

Asparagus is familiar as a seasonal vegetable – a summertime delicacy that is well worth attempting to grow in the vegetable garden. Its action as a medicinal plant will be familiar to most asparagus eaters, who will no doubt have noted its diuretic effect and the characteristic smell – caused by its breakdown to a substance called methylmercaptan – which it produces in the urine, often within a very few minutes of enjoying a bowl of spears.

Several species are used medicinally including *A. racemosus*, which is an important tonic herb (known as *shatavari*) in Ayurvedic medicine. The name *shatavari* means "who possesses a hundred husbands" and the herb is believed in India to have an extremely beneficial effect on the female reproductive organs. *Shatavari* is – predictably – recommended for menopausal problems and also for digestive and lung disorders. It is often eaten in a mixture with honey, milk and clarified butter.

Our more familiar Western vegetable – *A. officinalis* – has long been used as a cleansing herb for rheumatism and to support liver function. Asparagus has been promoted as a slimming aid by some producers of over-the-counter products, largely because of its diuretic and laxative action. It can help to disperse urinary stones and, as a good source of vitamins and minerals (including iron), it is ideal for debility and anaemia. Methylmercaptan can be irritant in cystitis, so it is best to avoid eating asparagus when suffering an attack; it also has a high purine content, so needs to be eaten in

moderation by gout sufferers. Asparagus soup should certainly be included regularly in the menu of convalescents and anyone prone to iron-deficiency anaemia.

Oats *Avena sativa*
Parts used: seeds, aerial parts
Actions: oatstraw – anti-depressant, restorative nerve tonic, diaphoretic; seeds – anti-depressant, restorative nerve tonic, nutritive; bran – anti-thrombotic, lowers cholesterol levels; fresh plant – anti-rheumatic in homoeopathic tincture

Oats – despite Dr Johnson's dismissal as "a grain which in England is generally given to horses, but in Scotland supports the people" – are one of the world's most important cereal crops, used as a staple food in northern Europe for centuries. Oats are sweet, nutritious and warming – ideal to combat a cold, damp, northern climate. They are rich in iron, zinc and manganese, so are also a good source of many vital minerals.

The plant is anti-depressant, a restorative nerve tonic and regarded as emotionally uplifting, so a bowl of porridge made from good-quality oatmeal is the ideal way to start the day. Extracts of the whole plant – the oatstraw – are generally used medicinally: the tincture is often combined with vervain for nervous problems, exhaustion and depression, emotional upsets associated with the menopause, or debility following illness.

The juice of fresh oats, pressed when still green, is similarly used as a nerve tonic. Oatstraw baths are used in folk medicine to counter rheumatic pains.

Oats *Avena sativa*

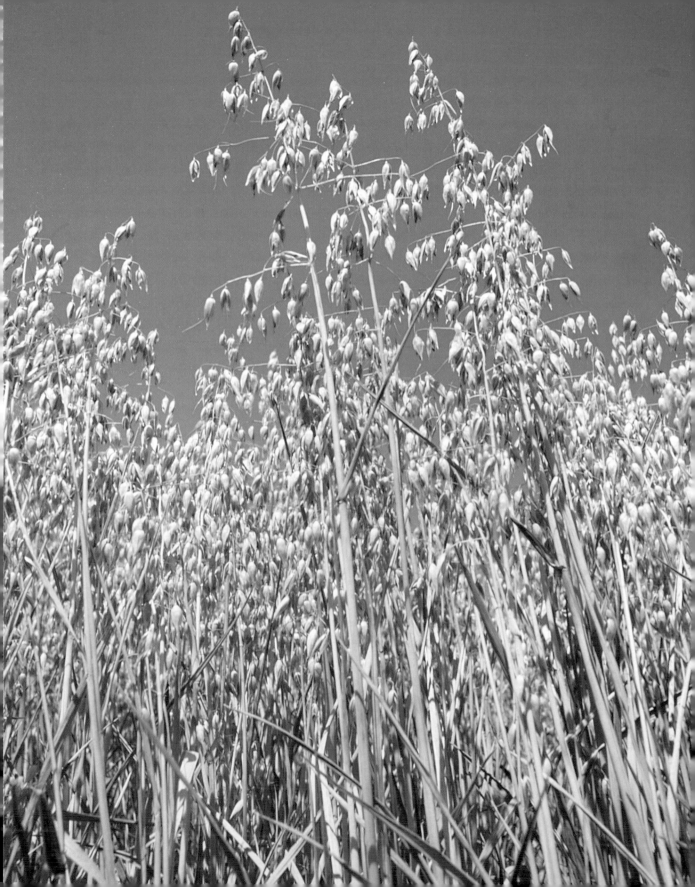

feet they can help to reduce over-all body temperature by dissipating heat. Use a tablespoon of mustard powder or seeds, preferably in a muslin bag, to a bowl of hot water and soak the feet for 10-15 minutes.

Both black and white mustard seeds are ground for use in pickles and sauces. They can usefully be made into hot infused oils (often combined with chili) for home use to make a warming rub for muscular stiffness, aches and pains.

Caution: Mustards can irritate the skin and prolonged use of poultices can lead to blistering.

Cabbage *Brassica oleracea*
Parts used: aerial parts
Actions: anti-inflammatory, anti-bacterial, anti-rheumatic, liver decongestant, tissue proliferant and healing

Jean Valnet, a notable contemporary French herbalist, has described cabbage as "the medicine of the poor" and it is probably one of the most widely used household remedies in folk tradition. The leaves have been used as anti-inflammatory poultices to relieve complaints ranging from arthritis to mastitis, while cabbage lotions were once a regular household standby for skin problems. Juices and infusions are used to treat a range of digestive problems including stomach ulcers.

The cabbage has been cultivated in the West since at least 400 BC, while in the second century AD the Greek herbalist Dioscorides considered it as a digestive remedy, joint tonic and cooling preparation for skin problems and fevers. Raw cabbage eaten before meat was reckoned to prevent drunkenness by over-indulgent Romans. In Germany sauerkraut, a fermented

cabbage mixture, is regarded as a preventative for cancer, rheumatism, gout and premature ageing.

The fresh leaves can be used directly on inflammations (simply soften them with a vegetable mallet and secure with a loose bandage or sticking plaster), while a useful lotion for acne can be made by combining cabbage leaves and distilled witch hazel in a food processor – chop enough cabbage leaves to fill about a third to a half of the processor, then cover them with witch hazel and blend to produce the right consistency. Cabbage juice is commercially available.

Tea *Camellia sinensis*
Part used: leaves
Actions: stimulant, anti-bacterial, anti-oxidant, astringent, diuretic, some varieties reduce cholesterol levels, anti-tumour properties reported in green teas

When tea was first introduced into Europe in the 17th century it was regarded not as an everyday drink but as a medicinal herb; numerous tea-house advertisements from the time extol the plant's virtues as a digestive remedy and cure for over-indulgence. Tea has been drunk in China since around 3000 BC when a mythical figure, Shen Nong – the "divine husbandman" – supposedly discovered its properties when a few leaves fell from an overhanging branch into a kettle of water he was boiling conveniently underneath.

The plant has a stimulating effect on the nervous system thanks to its caffeine-like alkaloids. Most of the tea drunk in the West is black tea made by fermenting

Clockwise from top left: tea *Camellia sinensis,* **chili** *Capsicum frutescens,* **lemon** *Citrus limonum,* **cinnamon** *Cinnamomum zeylanicum*

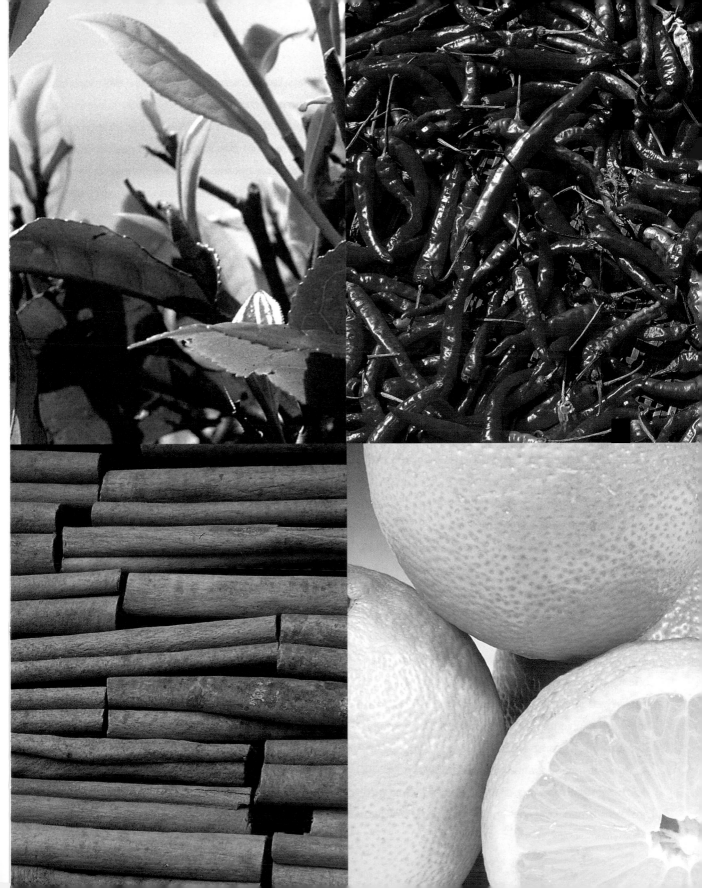

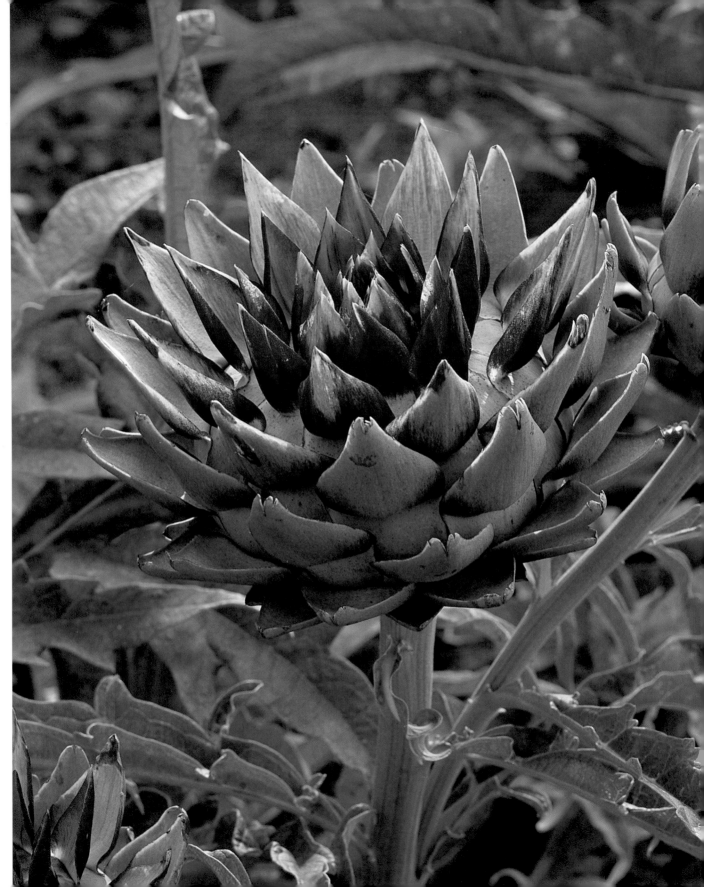

Artichoke *Cynara cardunculus* (Scolymus Group)

Part used: flower heads

Actions: alterative, bile stimulant, digestive stimulant, diuretic, heart tonic, laxative, liver tonic

Globe artichokes have been regarded as a delicacy since the days of Theophrastus in the fourth century BC: he tells us that the plant grew in Sicily and while good to eat, must be enjoyed fresh since – unlike many other vegetables – it could not be pickled in brine (a favourite Greek method of storing winter vegetables).

The edible part is actually the flower head and until recently this bitter-tasting vegetable was regarded as little more than a mild digestive stimulant. However, we now know that cynarin, found in the plant, can stimulate bile flow and also has a protective action on the liver, encouraging regeneration and repair. It is also considered a potent remedy for gall bladder problems, with artichoke juice used to ease the symptoms of nausea, pain and dyspepsia associated with poor gall bladder function. Researchers have also found that globe artichoke can help to lower blood cholesterol levels, possibly associated with the healing effect it has on fatty degeneration of the liver.

As well as these important actions, artichokes are diuretic and will encourage uric acid excretion, so may be supportive for gout sufferers; they are also cleansing and energising. Eating artichokes can be helpful in convalescence, arthritic disorders and whenever there are liver or gall bladder problems. Artichoke juice and syrup are both available commercially, or you can simply eat artichokes as a vegetable.

Artichoke *Cynara cardunculus*

The globe artichoke should not be confused with Jerusalem artichoke (*Helianthus tuberosus*), a North American relative of the sunflower cultivated for its tuberous roots, which are eaten as a vegetable. The plant was brought to Europe at the end of the 16th century and was known as "potatoes of Canada". The tubers are rich in a starch called inulin, which does not break down in the digestive process to form glucose, so Jerusalem artichokes make an ideal food for diabetes sufferers. Although little used medicinally, Jerusalem artichokes can be helpful as a digestive stimulant and in constipation.

Carrot *Daucus carota* subsp. *sativus*

Parts used: root, aerial parts, oil

Actions: anti-anaemic, cleansing, digestive tonic, diuretic, immune stimulant, nutrient, tonic

The wild carrot (*D. carota*), also known as Queen Anne's lace, is a popular medicinal herb widely used as a diuretic and carminative and given for urinary stones, cystitis and gout. Wild carrot root is white and inedible but the more familiar orange vegetable also has a number of valuable properties.

The carrot has been cultivated in most parts of Europe and North Africa since ancient times and, until the introduction of the potato from North America, it was widely eaten as a staple food. It is rich in a substance called *beta*-carotene, which is converted into Vitamin A in the body, and is traditionally said to improve the eyesight – Vitamin A is essential for good night vision. Carrots are also a good source of Vitamins B and C, and of several minerals including iron, potassium and calcium.

As well as being highly nutritious, carrots are believed to stimulate the immune system and in recent years have been regarded as an important addition to anti-cancer diets; many nutritionists suggest that regular consumption of carrots can have a preventive effect. Carrots and carrot juice are also recommended as a readily digestible food source in debility and convalescence and for anaemia, diarrhoea, chest problems (including chronic bronchitis), rheumatism, gout, constipation, intestinal worms and digestive upsets.

Externally they can be used for skin disorders – including eczema – and abscesses: both the juice and carrot oil (commercially available and often included in cosmetic anti-wrinkle products) are used. Research also suggests that *beta*-carotene can provide some protection from the sun's ultra-violet rays, so carrot is often suggested by beauticians as a useful supplement before sunbathing.

Caution: Vitamin A is one of the few vitamins that can be extremely toxic in large doses, affecting the liver and turning the skin a yellow colour; however, *beta*-carotene is believed to be rather safer as most of the surplus is excreted.

Fig *Ficus carica*
Part used: fruit
Actions: diuretic, emollient, laxative, nutrient

Fig syrup has been used as a household standby for constipation since the days of the Pharaohs. An ancient Egyptian papyrus dating from 1500 BC gives a recipe based on figs soaked overnight in "sweet beer" which had to be drunk "often". The Egyptians also regarded the fig as a heart remedy and recommended it to combat lung disease – possibly based on a Doctrine of Signatures theory as the rounded, ripe fig vaguely resembles these organs.

The fig originated in Asia Minor but has been grown in Western Europe since Roman times: the French king Charlemagne encouraged fig growing in the ninth century and the tree is still a common sight in rural French gardens.

The fruits have a laxative effect and are often used combined with senna (*Senna alexandrina*). Externally fig poultices were once applied to boils and varicose ulcers, and the fruit is also considered as a demulcent to soothe irritated tissues such as in sore throats, coughs and bronchial problems.

Eating fresh or dried figs for breakfast is a pleasant way to counter any tendency to habitual constipation.

Strawberry *Fragaria vesca*
Parts used: fruit, leaves
Actions: astringent, wound herb, diuretic, laxative, liver tonic, cleansing

Strawberries have been cultivated in Britain since at least the 10th century and were valued as both a food and a healing remedy. The leaves are mildly astringent and diuretic and are often added to herbal tea blends: they can be helpful for diarrhoea and digestive upsets.

The root was once a popular household remedy for diarrhoea and the stalks were used for wounds – Culpeper declared it "singularly good for the healing of many ills".

Strawberry *Fragaria vesca*

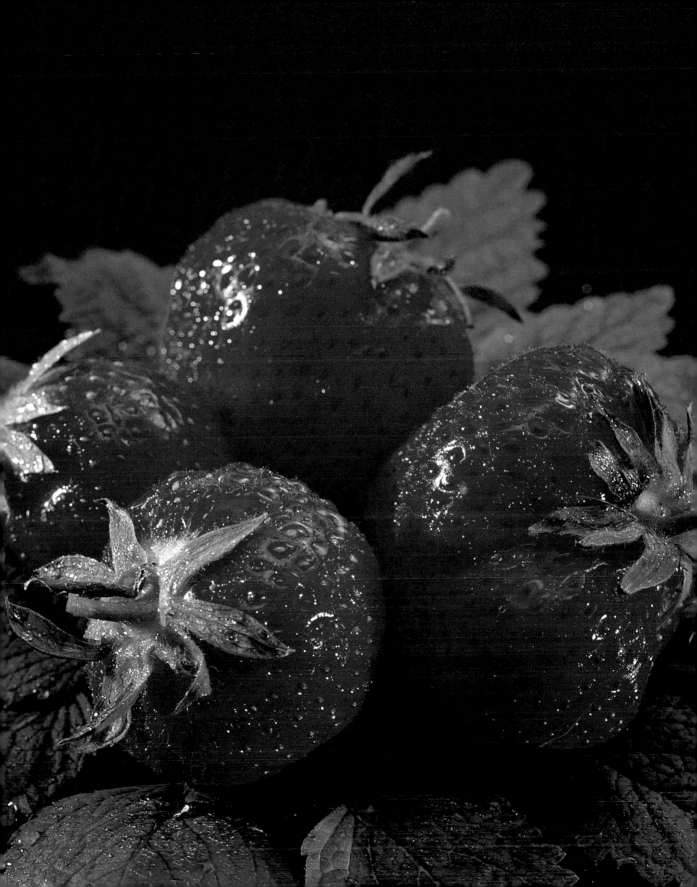

Pear *Pyrus communis*

Part used: fruit

Actions: astringent, cleansing, digestive tonic, diuretic, laxative, sedative

Like many fruits, pears were regarded in Galenical medicine as "colde" with a "binding quality". William Turner recommended a broth of dried pears as a remedy for diarrhoea, while the juice was reckoned to be "good for the biting of venomous beasts". Turner also added that "pears are good for the stomach and quench thirst if they be taken in meat".

We tend to consider pears as more suitable for constipation, but as with apples much depends on ripeness and how the fruit has been prepared, as the properties can vary significantly – or to quote from Turner again: "Raw pears burden the stomach, but roasted or sodden relieve and lighten the stomach."

The pear's cleansing characteristics make it especially suitable in rheumatism and arthritis and the fruit is also rich in vitamins and minerals (including iron, phosphorus and calcium), so can be helpful in debility, convalescence or iron-deficient anaemia.

Gerard recommended hot perry (a pear-based alternative to cider) for stomach chills, while in France pear juice before meals is believed to help the digestion. Try warm pear juice for stomach upsets or eat two or three fresh pears a day if constipation is a habitual problem.

Potato *Solanum tuberosum*

Part used: tuber

Actions: antispasmodic, mild anodyne, digestive remedy, diuretic, emollient, nutrient

Potatoes belong to the same family as deadly nightshade and henbane and, like these highly toxic herbs, contain poisonous alkaloids. Solanine, found in potato skin, has the same sort of antispasmodic properties as atropine (found in deadly nightshade) and in large quantities would be equally fatal. Indeed, if the potato was discovered today scientists would probably condemn it as not safe for human consumption.

Fortunately potatoes were introduced into Europe in a more adventurous age: they were brought to Spain from Peru in 1530 and Sir Walter Raleigh is credited with planting the first potatoes in Britain during the days of Elizabeth I. It took around 200 years for the potato to supplant bread, barley and carrots as the main staple in our diet – partly because of its association with the nightshade family. Tomatoes – another close relative – suffered a similar fate and were regarded as toxic and purely ornamental until well into the 18th century.

Today, potatoes are possibly the most important source of Vitamin C in the average British diet. They are also rich in B-complex vitamins (including B_1, B_5, B_6 and folic acid) and contain several minerals, including iron, calcium, manganese, magnesium and phosphorus.

In the days when every housewife knew how to make a poultice, mashed potato was the preferred choice of many of them and was widely applied to just about every ache, pain and inflammation. As well as being an important food source, potato juice is a useful addition to the medicine chest. It can be helpful for relieving digestive problems associated with excessive stomach acid – including indigestion, gastritis and peptic

Clockwise from top left: potato *Solanum tuberosum;* **bilberry** *Vaccinium myrtillus;* **ginger** *Zingiber officinale;* **grape** *Vitis vinifera*

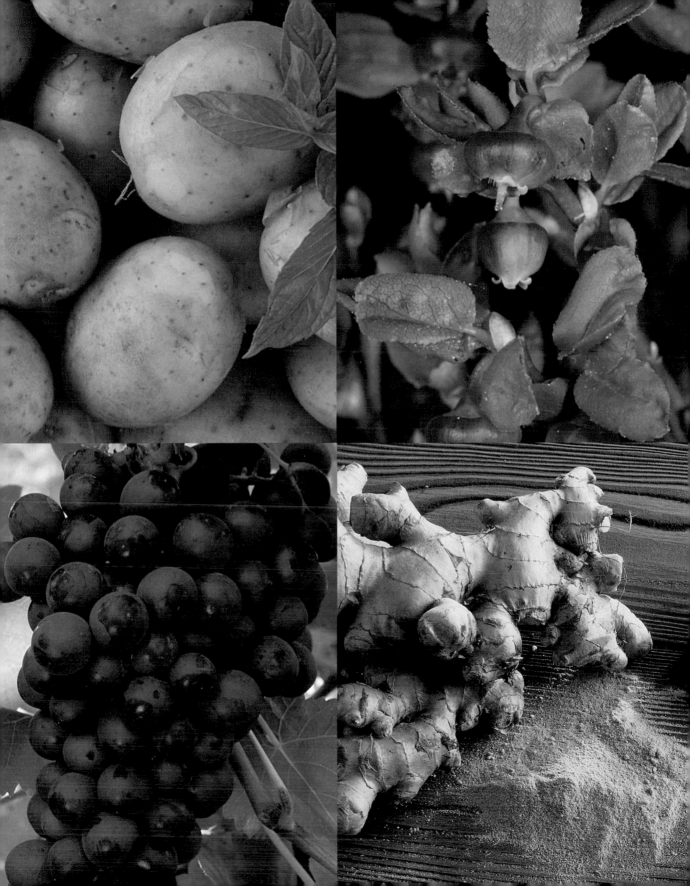

ulcers – and is a good liver remedy which can also be helpful for bile stones and gall bladder problems.

Externally raw potato can be used to soothe skin inflammations. It has long been regarded as a folk remedy for burns and scalds (try grated potato mixed with vegetable oil), but the tradition is now being adopted by orthodox medicine thanks to some pioneering work by burns specialists in India using potato peelings.

Cloves *Syzygium aromaticum*
Part used: flower buds
Actions: mild anaesthetic, anodyne, anti-emetic, antiseptic, antispasmodic, carminative, warming stimulant

Cloves have been used for flavouring for around 2000 years and were known in Roman times as an exotic spice. The Chinese have used them medicinally since around 600 AD, regarding them as a kidney tonic, increasing *yang* energy and ideal for treating impotence.

Clove oil is available from pharmacies and is useful as an emergency first-aid remedy for toothache (put a few drops on a cotton-wool swab and place on the gum nearest to the aching tooth). Cloves are often included in "herbal" toothpastes and dental preparations.

Cloves are useful for disguising the taste of more unpleasant herbs, so a couple added to a herbal mixture for stomach upsets or chills can often make the brew rather more palatable.

In many parts of the East, clove oil is also used as an abdominal massage during labour to encourage contractions and ease pain. While this is certainly not something the novice should attempt, drinking teas flavoured with plenty of cloves during the second stage of labour can help to ease childbirth pains.

Caution: Cloves should be reserved for labour and child-birth and not taken earlier in pregnancy.

Wheat *Triticum* spp.
Parts used: seeds, aerial parts
Actions: anti-oxidant, diuretic, laxative, tonic

Wheat is one of our oldest cereal crops, cultivated in Mesopotamia more than 10,000 years ago and still the major staple for millions of Europeans. It is highly nutritious and the whole grains are rich in Vitamins A, B-complex, D and E while wheatgerm oil is an even better source of Vitamin E than the grain and contains a number of essential fatty acids. Commercial over-processing means that many of these nutrients are lost from the bread we eat and are often artificially added at the production stage – using wholemeal and organic flours is always advisable.

Although primarily regarded as a nutrient, wheat has its medicinal uses as well. Wheat bran is irritant on the gut and can be helpful for constipation – although excessive use can lead to long-term damage and increase the risk of diverticulitis. Wheatgerm, because of its Vitamin E component, is a good anti-oxidant, so can counter the effect of ageing on the body's cells. It can also be helpful for menstrual problems and increase fertility.

Externally wheat bran can be used like oatmeal as a facial scrub, while bread poultices have long been a favourite folk remedy for drawing splinters and boils and also reducing swellings and inflammation.

Wheatgrass can be made by sprouting wheat grains on blotting paper in the kitchen and is a good source of chlorophyll and many enzymes. Cut the grass after three or four days, when it is around 5 cm high, and add to salads as a good source of trace elements.

Bilberry *Vaccinium myrtillus*
Parts used: leaves, fruit
Actions: antiseptic, anti-emetic, astringent, hypoglycaemic, tonic

Although bilberries – and their close relatives like cowberries (*V. vitis-idaea*), cranberries (*V. oxycoccos*) and farkleberries (*V. arboreum*) – were once regularly used as medicinal herbs, they have fallen from favour in recent years. Fruits of all four plants are rich in Vitamin C, highly astringent – due to their tannin content – and anti-bacterial. These culinary berries are closely related to bearberry (*Arctostaphylos uva-ursi*), an important urinary antiseptic, and recent work has highlighted the use of cranberry juice as an effective remedy for recurrent cystitis.

Elizabethan apothecaries used to make a syrup of the berries with honey, called rob, which was used as a remedy for diarrhoea. In large quantities, however, the berries have a laxative effect, so make an extremely palatable remedy for constipation.

Externally bilberries have been used in salves and ointments for piles, burns and skin complaints. Recent research has shown that the leaves, taken internally, will also reduce blood-sugar levels, so make a useful support for late-onset diabetes that is under dietary control, and there have been some suggestions that bilberry leaves can encourage insulin production.

The berries can be eaten stewed or fresh for digestive problems: the German herbalist, Dr Rudolf Weiss, recommended cooked bilberry topped with cheesecake for diarrhoea, as soft white cheese also has anti-diarrhoeic effects.

Grape *Vitis vinifera*
Parts used: fruit, leaves
Actions: astringent, anti-inflammatory, bile stimulant, cleansing, diuretic, laxative, liver stimulant, nerve and muscle tonic

Both vine leaves and grapes have been used in herbal medicine, while there is also increasing evidence that wine can have a beneficial effect on the heart and circulation – something the French have argued for years.

Vine leaves have been used to improve circulation and control bleeding. Ointments made from vine leaves are still used to relieve the discomfort of varicose veins and vine leaf tea can be used as a gargle for sore throats and a mouth wash for inflamed gums.

Among the numerous properties with which the grape is credited are bile stimulating and general liver cleansing. Grapes are also regarded as a good tonic food, helping to raise energy levels – hence their popularity with hospital visitors and in convalescence. Grape juice is often recommended as a key component in detoxification programmes and in chronic illness including cancer and severe arthritis, while eating grapes (fresh, or dried as raisins and sultanas) can be helpful for constipation and a sluggish digestion.

Wine is now known to help reduce cholesterol levels and provide some protection from heart disease – in moderation, of course – although some French authorities, such as Dr M. Maury, recommend various types of wine for just about every ailment from acidosis (try Pouilly-Fuissé) to urticaria (a Médoc or Côtes de Ventoux).

Ginger *Zingiber officinale*

Part used: root

Actions: anti-emetic, antiseptic, antispasmodic, carminative, circulatory stimulant, diaphoretic, expectorant, peripheral vasodilator; topically – rubefacient

Ginger originates from tropical Asia, but spread to Europe in ancient times: it is mentioned by the Romans, listed in some of the earliest Chinese herbals, regarded in Ayurvedic medicine as a universal medicine, and was introduced by the Spaniards to America where it is now cultivated extensively in the West Indies.

The plant is useful for controlling nausea and coughing. It has a pungent, aromatic flavour and is widely used as a commercial flavouring. Gerard described the fresh root as "hot and moist and provoking venerie" and laments his inability to grow the plant in his London garden. As a hot, dry herb it was used to warm the stomach and dispel chills. In the 18th century ginger was added to many remedies to modify their action and reduce the irritant effects on the stomach or, as Henry Barham put it in 1794, to "taketh away their malice" – a technique still practised in China, where ginger is cooked with such potentially poisonous plants as monkshood to reduce toxicity.

Fresh ginger from the greengrocer can be made into a warming tea for colds and chills (simply simmer a few slices in water as a decoction) or add a pinch of powdered ginger to other herb teas. Ginger oil is used in external remedies to encourage blood flow to ease muscular stiffness, aches and pains.

In Chinese medicine fresh and dried root are regarded rather differently, with the dried believed to be helpful for abdominal pain and diarrhoea and the fresh considered more suitable for treating feverish chills, coughs and vomiting.

As a remedy for nausea, ginger is ideal for travel sickness and has been successfully tested in clinical trials for very severe morning sickness in pregnancy (a typical dose is 1 g, three times a day). Ginger in capsules is ideal but ginger biscuits or ginger beer can also prove effective – especially with children. A hot infused oil made with ginger is a home-made alternative to the distilled essential oil.

helpful **houseplants**

We can also make use of the numerous exotic potted plants which are now available from nurseries and garden centres for home cultivation – both as medicinal remedies and generally to help improve the environment.

Plants have been grown in houses for centuries, sometimes for decoration but originally to serve more practical functions. The ancient Egyptians grew boswellia trees in tubs in palace courtyards as a source of frankincense, while the perfumed geraniums brought back to Europe from South Africa in the 17th century soon became popular for scenting rooms. Modern research has revealed an even more useful property for houseplants – many of them suck polluting chemicals from the atmosphere, breaking them down into harmless substances. Growing houseplants in town centre offices or inner city homes can really make the environment healthier for people who live and work there.

Philodendron spp., spider plants (*Chlorophytum elatum*), azaleas and weeping figs (*Ficus benjamina*) are all efficient at removing formaldehyde – a pollutant produced by some modern building materials as well as floor coverings, foam insulation and cleaning agents and also found in cigarette smoke and natural gas – from the atmosphere, while the common ivy (*Hedera helix*) rapidly clears benzene contained in some car exhaust fumes and the peace lily or white flag (*Spathiphyllum* spp.) soaks up trichloroethylene from dry cleaning fluid with enthusiasm.

Recent work has also focused on yuccas, which absorb urea from the atmosphere, welcoming it as a source of nitrogen. The habit makes the plant ideal for growing in lavatories to help reduce smells.

Also worth growing in pots indoors are:

Aloe vera – which also absorbs atmospheric pollutants (see page 83).

Dendrobium nobile orchids, commonly grown as houseplants in Europe, but the stems are used in Chinese medicine for feverish colds and dry coughs.

Passion flower (see page 67) can be grown outside in warm areas; otherwise keep it as a conservatory or indoor climber and use the leaves in teas for insomnia.

The florist's chrysanthemum (*Chrysanthemum morifolium*) is another Chinese medicinal plant. The flowers are known as *Ju Hua* and are used for liver and high blood pressure remedies. They are popular as a tea in China – sold Western-style in ready-made drinks and tea bags – but they do need to be steamed before use to reduce the bitter taste.

wildflower **remedies**

The sight of the village "herb wife" gathering her medicines from fields and hedges to brew into healing potions over the cottage fire is an image which probably stopped being commonplace in Britain more than 150 years ago. The Industrial Revolution and Enclosure Acts changed rural life dramatically and many of the old healing skills were lost. When Dr William Withering began experimenting with Mrs Hutton's cure for dropsy in 1775 – work which eventually led to the discovery of the heart drug digitoxin – Mrs Hutton was already something of an anachronism.

Today it is not unusual for popular herbals to give step-by-step instructions for making herb teas: with so many people used to tea-bags or "instant" varieties, the idea of steeping leaves in a pot seems to be something that has now to be taught. Equally the very thought of gathering a few sprigs from the roadside or garden and using them to make something to drink, leaves many people convinced that a highly toxic brew will inevitably be produced. Their concerns can sometimes be justified – excessive use of chemical sprays in agriculture can produce many poisonous residues on otherwise perfectly safe leaves.

This same over-enthusiasm for weedkillers and pesticides, combined with enthusiastic trimming by local authorities, means that many of our once-common field and woodland flowers are now rare and it can be extremely difficult to find a natural source of herbs like marsh woundwort and bear's breech. Others, such as yarrow, chickweed, St John's wort and shepherd's purse do remain extremely common, and these plants can provide valuable emergency first-aid treatments when far from home. Fresh crushed leaves, rinsed in fresh water (if there is any nearby) to remove dust and soil, can be ideal to stop bleeding or to wrap around a sprained joint as a make-shift poultice.

In recent years in Europe the "set aside" policy for agricultural land has encouraged a return of some wild flowers, but as the rules demand cutting set aside land periodically to keep it in reasonable agricultural condition, only the fastest growing weeds have a chance to prosper. Set aside can, however, be a good source of yellow dock, agrimony and common mallow. Many other hedgerow herbs can be grown in gardens, and wild flower seeds are readily available. Although these are native European plants, for historical reasons they have also been widely cultivated in other parts of the world, notably Australia and New Zealand. Several of the plants listed in this section can be invasive weeds (especially when grown outside Europe), so take care if you plan to introduce them into the garden!

Correct identification is, of course, important – especially where toxic plants are concerned. Foxglove when not in flower can easily be mistaken for comfrey, for example. It is always much easier to identify plants when they are flowering and since most can be collected then, this reduces the risks of error. Several plants can be difficult to find at certain times of the year: it is useful, for example, to note any coltsfoot plants in summer when the leaves are obvious so that the flowers – which are more difficult to spot – can be collected the following spring. When gathering plants in the wild try to choose specimens away from busy roads to limit pollution from petrol and diesel fumes and avoid areas close to farmland where chemical sprays may have been used.

Brief botanical descriptions and illustrations are given for all the plants in this section: flowering times given are average for northern Europe and similar temperate climates.

For an explanation of any unfamiliar terms, on the following pages, consult the glossary on pages 183-185; for advice on typical dosages and on preparing your own remedies, see pages 24-40.

Bear's breech *Acanthus mollis*

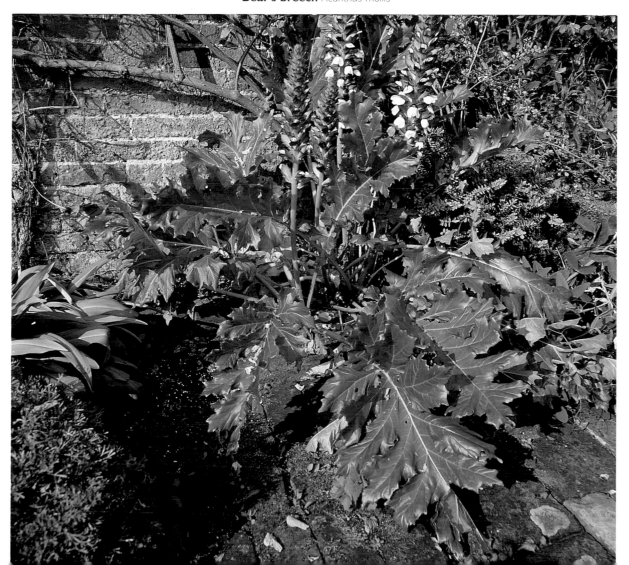

Bear's breech *Acanthus mollis*

Description: a hardy perennial growing to 150 cm with striking broad glossy, dark-green, pinnate leaves. The flower spikes bear white, pale blue or pale purple tube-shaped flowers with a three-lobed lip, appearing in late summer and lasting until early autumn.

Part used: leaves, gathered before flowering

Actions: bile stimulant, demulcent, mild laxative, vulnerary

The plant originates from the Steppes of Asia but has long been grown in Mediterranean areas and was introduced into Britain in the Middle Ages. Bear's breech was once common in the West Country, although it is now comparatively rare in the wild but is often grown as a garden plant.

Its botanical name comes from the Greek *akanthos* meaning "thorn flowers" and acanthus leaves are a common motif in ancient Greek sculpture and decoration – they are the inspiration for the classic design of Corinthian columns.

The herb is rich in mucilage and tannins and was traditionally used as a soothing wound herb. Crushed leaves, soaked in cold water, were made into poultices for gout or used to ease burns and scalds. As a mild laxative and bile stimulant, the juice was traditionally used as a digestive tonic to improve appetite and cleanse the liver. "Acanthus tea" was also once recommended for bladder inflammations.

Yarrow *Achillea millefolium*

Description: a perennial herb with distinctive feathery leaves and tiny white flowers in clusters appearing throughout the summer and autumn.

Parts used: leaves collected throughout the growing season; flowers gathered when in full bloom

Yarrow *Achillea millefolium*

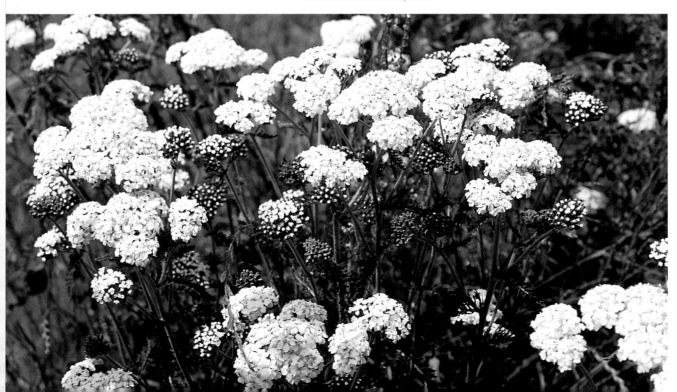

Actions: anti-inflammatory, antispasmodic, astringent, bitter, carminative, diaphoretic, digestive tonic, diuretic, febrifuge, hypotensive, peripheral vasodilator, styptic, urinary antiseptic

A common meadow herb, yarrow's folk name – nosebleed – confirms its traditional first-aid use as an emergency styptic: simply insert a couple of fresh leaves into the nostril and the feathery leaves provide an ideal encouragement for clotting.

Yarrow relaxes the peripheral blood vessels, so can help to reduce high blood pressure and it is also cooling in fevers. Like chamomile flowers, yarrow flowers contain anti-allergenic compounds which are activated by hot water or steam, so are found only in infusions and the distilled essential oil, not in the tincture or fresh plant. Yarrow tea can be helpful for colds, influenza, hay fever and catarrh and can also be added to urinary remedies.

The plant was once used in divination and folk rituals still associate it with prediction (generally by identifying future husbands): the same tradition persists in China where yarrow stalks are used with the *I Ching*. In Germany and Nordic countries yarrow was once used instead of hops in beer making. The oil is available commercially, and is anti-inflammatory and anti-allergenic. It can be used in steam inhalations for hay fever and chest rubs for colds and catarrh.

Caution: Yarrow should be avoided in pregnancy as it is a uterine stimulant. The fresh herb can sometimes cause contact dermatitis and, in rare cases, prolonged use may increase the skin's photosensitivity.

Agrimony *Agrimonia eupatoria*

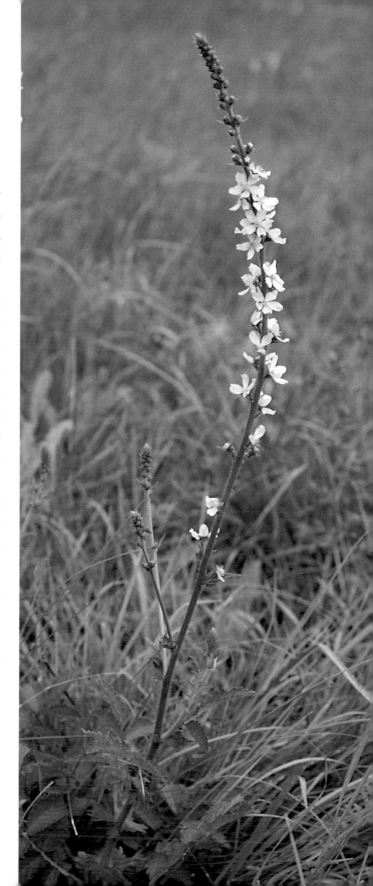

Agrimony *Agrimonia eupatoria*

Description: an erect perennial herb growing to 60 cm in height with downy, serrated leaves in three to five pairs, larger at the base (where they may be 20 cm long) and getting smaller further up the stem. Five-petalled yellow flowers grow on tall flower spikes flowering from the bottom of the stem upwards, throughout the summer.

Parts used: aerial parts gathered in summer while flowering but before too many burr-like seed heads have formed

Actions: astringent, bitter digestive tonic, bile stimulant, diuretic, hepatic, styptic, vulnerary

The tall yellow flower spikes of agrimony can still be seen at roadsides in high summer, giving the plant its old common name of "church steeples". The herb, like all members of the rose family, is strongly astringent; writing in the second century AD, Dioscorides recommended it to stop bleeding and for dysentery.

The *eupatoria* part of the name is reputedly derived from Mithridates Eupator, an ancient king of Pontus and renowned herbalist. Since Saxon times agrimony has been used as a wound-herb and in the 15th century was the prime ingredient of arquebasade water – a battlefield remedy for early gunshot wounds.

It is still used for diarrhoea and is suitably gentle for children and babies – nursing mothers can take agrimony infusion as a means of dosing their babies via breast milk. Drink a cup of a weak infusion (15 g of herb to 500 ml of water) two hours before feeds up to four times a day.

Agrimony is a bitter herb that will stimulate bile flow and has a tonic effect on the digestion. It can be useful for those prone to food allergies, helping them to absorb foods more easily while repairing damage to the gut caused by allergens. It also has a high silica content – hence its action as a tissue healer. As a diuretic it is sometimes included in remedies for cystitis and other urinary problems and combines well with imported herbs like buchu (see page 49).

Jack-by-the-hedge *Alliaria petiolata*

Description: a biennial with a distinctive garlic smell, bright green rounded leaves and small white flowers in spring and summer. Grows up to 120 cm in height.

Part used: leaves, collected during flowering

Actions: antiseptic, anti-inflammatory, diuretic, expectorant, vulnerary

Garlic mustard is an alternative and very apt name for this common hedgerow plant which is characterised by the garlic smell obtained when the leaves are crushed. It makes a useful spicy addition to salads and can also be cooked to produce a mild garlic-flavoured sauce.

The plant has a long medical history and was once known as *Alliaria officinalis* – suggesting that it was once listed in official pharmacopoeia. Like garlic it contains various sulphur compounds as well as sinigrin – found in other members of the cabbage family – which account for its smell.

Poultices of Jack-by-the-hedge were once used for skin sores and cuts, applied hot to rheumatic aches and pains, or for neuralgia. It was a popular wound herb also used for digestive problems.

Clockwise from top left: Jack-by-the-hedge
Alliaria petiolata, **ramsons** *Allium ursinum*, **burdock**
Arctium lappa, **marshmallow** *Althaea officinalis*

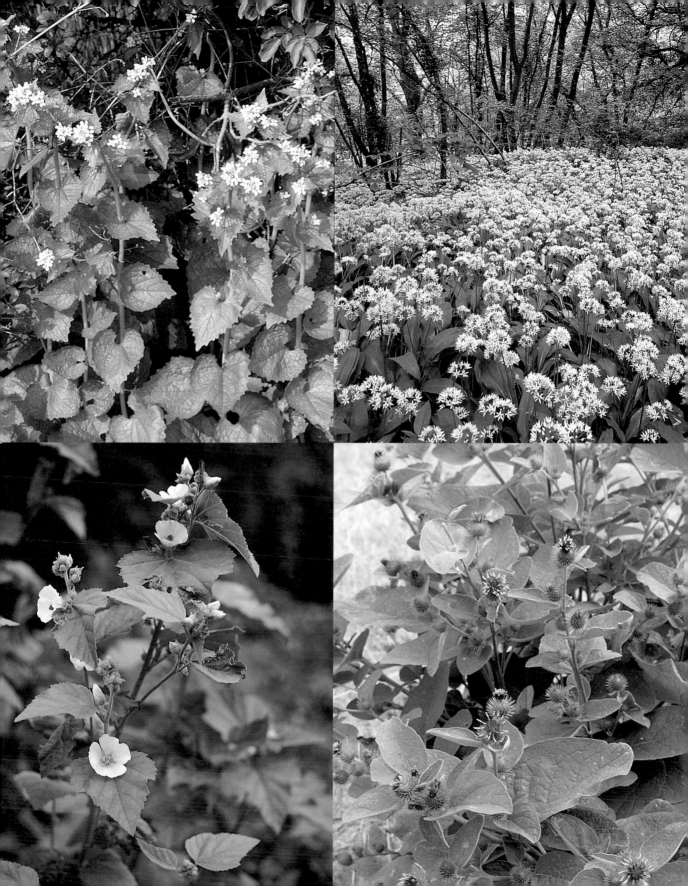

William Turner included it as "saucealone" in the third part of his *New Herball* – published in 1568 – suggesting that it was "hot in the second degree after the rules of Galen" and recommending it for "them that have a cold stomach…but not good for them that…have hot blood or be disposed to the headache".

As well as using the plant to spice up seasonal salads, it is well worth trying as a tea for colds and chills; it can also make a warming drink (or be used in sauces) for rheumatic sufferers.

Ramsons *Allium ursinum*

Description: a garlic-scented perennial growing from a white bulb with elliptical leaves up to 30 cm long and clusters of white, six-petalled, star-like flowers in early to midsummer.

Parts used: whole plant gathered while flowering, or leaves collected after flowering

Actions: very similar to garlic (see page 83) – anti-bacterial, anti-fungal, diaphoretic, hypotensive, reduces cholesterol levels

Ramsons grow wild throughout Europe adding a wonderful garlicky scent to spring woodlands. The plant has been used in folk medicine since Greek times much as cultivated garlic has been – as a remedy for infections, chest complaints and digestive disorders, as well as being used as a blood purifier and spring tonic. The common name derives from *hramson* which was Old English for "wild garlic" and the plant is also known as bear's garlic or broad-leaved garlic.

Like garlic it also helps reduce blood cholesterol levels and has been used to treat high blood pressure caused by atherosclerosis. As a strongly anti-bacterial and anti-fungal plant, it is also used to treat yeast-related infections helping to normalise the gut flora.

Ramsons are rather milder in flavour than ordinary garlic and may be better tolerated by those with sensitive stomachs. The leaves can be chopped and added to salads.

Marshmallow *Althaea officinalis*

Description: an erect, sturdy perennial with soft, downy, round to ovate leaves and large, pale pink flowers in the axils in summer. The plant grows to around 120 cm in height and prefers damp, marshy places.

Parts used: leaves collected before flowering, root collected in the autumn and flowers when in bloom

Actions: alterative, anti-tussive, demulcent, diuretic, emollient, vulnerary

Marshmallow grows in damp, sunny places and is a close relative of the familiar garden hollyhock. The plant produces a sweet-tasting, highly mucilaginous root that is rich in sugars and is eaten as a foodstuff in many parts of the world – writing in the 1930s, the herbalist Maud Grieve recommended them boiled first and then fried with onions and butter. The sugars help to make marsh-mallow very soothing and demulcent (softening) and the plant is widely used to calm inflamed mucous membranes especially of the lungs and digestive system – so it can be helpful for gastritis, heartburn and other inflammations.

The botanical name comes from a Greek word, *altho*, meaning "to heal" and the plants have certainly been used medicinally since ancient Egyptian times. The whole herb is also an expectorant, so is ideal for irritating coughs.

The leaves and flowers are also used medicinally: at one time the flowers were collected separately and made into cough syrups, although these days commercial cultivation means that all the aerial parts tend to be combined. The leaves have also been cooked as a vegetable while the young tips can be added to salads. Marshmallow root and leaves are diuretic, so make a soothing addition to cystitis remedies.

Externally the plant is equally valuable and healing. It can be made into ointments for various sores and skin problems and, combined with slippery elm, it makes a good drawing ointment for splinters and boils. The root or leaves can easily be made into a syrup, providing a valuable standby for winter coughs.

Burdock *Arctium lappa*

Description: a tall biennial herb growing to 200 cm with large dock-like leaves, ovate to heart-shaped, with round purple flowers blooming from early summer to early autumn. The seed heads form characteristic burrs with hooked tips.

Parts used: leaves collected during the flowering season, second-year roots lifted in autumn

Actions: alterative, antibiotic, diaphoretic, diuretic, mild laxative

It is still possible to find traditional "dandelion and burdock" cordials on supermarket shelves – although nowadays the product is likely to be promoted as a pleasant drink rather than a cleansing herbal remedy for skin problems and arthritis.

The herb commonly grows wild in Europe and parts of Asia and is familiar for its hooked burrs which get caught in clothing and animal fur – a property reflected in the botanical name, derived from the Greek *arctium* meaning "bear", suggesting rough-coated fruits, and *lappa*, which means "to seize".

As one might expect from a traditional cleansing herb, it is a mild laxative and diuretic, useful where a sluggish digestion is contributing to a build-up of toxins.

Although not used in the West, the seeds are a traditional China remedy for feverish colds – an action which modern research confirms with the identification of strong anti-microbial activity in the seeds. They will also help to lower blood sugar levels, so could be useful in the management of late-onset diabetes.

Burdock produces a long tap root in its second year: this is cultivated as a vegetable (known as *gobo*) in Japan. Western herbalists tend to regard the root as more potent than the leaf and it is used in a number of over-the-counter remedies, largely for skin and rheumatic complaints. Burdock is often combined with yellow dock in skin remedies. The leaves can be taken in infusion while the root and seeds are best added to decoctions.

Daisy *Bellis perennis*

Description: low-growing perennial with a basal rosette of oval leaves and numerous distinctive white and yellow flowers often with pink tinge to the petals. It blooms from spring to late autumn.

Parts used: aerial parts, gathered during flowering

Actions: antispasmodic, astringent, expectorant, possibly anti-viral, relieves muscle pains

One of the old names for daisy was bruisewort – a reference to its popular use in ointments and poultices for bruises. The botanical name comes from the Latin

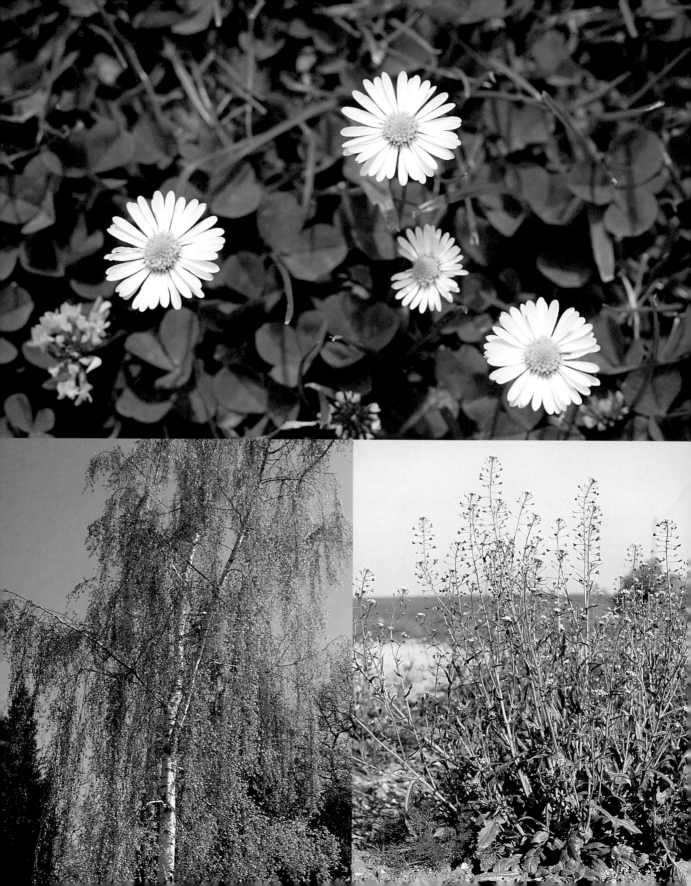

bellus – pretty – and its English name is a corruption of "day's eye": daisy flowers open only in sunshine and will tuck their heads away as dusk falls.

The herb was once popular for wounds, while the leaves were used in poultices or made into an infusion to drink for lumbago, stiff neck or other aches and pains. Gerard suggests pounding fresh daisies with unsalted butter as a simple ointment for all sorts of pains, adding that "…they worke more effectually if mallowes be added thereto".

He also suggests putting drops of daisy juice into the nostrils to clear catarrh and migraine while "the same given to little dogs with milke, keepeth them from growing great" – which provides an interesting insight into how Elizabethans regarded their pets.

A decoction of the root was used as a cleansing remedy for skin problems and could also be taken for respiratory complaints and liver disorders, while chewing fresh leaves is a traditional folk cure for mouth ulcers. The leaves also contain saponins and have been used in cough remedies.

Birch *Betula pendula*
Description: a slender, short-lived tree, with drooping branches and silvery-white bark which tends to peel off easily. Male and female catkins appear in spring with winged nutlets in autumn.
Parts used: leaves, collected in summer; bark and sap collected in autumn.
Actions: anti-inflammatory, astringent, bitter, bile stimulant, diuretic

Top: daisy *Bellis perennis;* **bottom left: birch** *Betula pendula;* **bottom right: shepherd's purse** *Capsella bursa-pastoris*

Birch is highly regarded as a medicinal plant in many areas of Northern Europe – especially Russia and Scandinavia where it is a favourite for treating rheumatism, gout and arthritis. The tree contains salicylates, which accounts for its anti-inflammatory and anti-rheumatic action.

Both leaves and bark can be used in teas to relieve aches and pains and are also suitably astringent for use in mouth washes and gargles for sore gums, mouth ulcers and sore throats. As a diuretic the plant can also be helpful in cystitis and is often used with stinging nettles as a general cleanser and detoxificant for chronic conditions.

The sap can be collected as it falls back in the autumn by "tapping" the tree: make a hole through the bark and collect the large amounts of sap it produces in a bucket. Remember to stop up the hole after taking the sap to prevent the tree from bleeding to death. This sap can then be added to internal remedies for rheumatism or used to make birch wine. An oil, distilled from the bark and known as birch tar oil, is used in ointments or lotions for psoriasis and eczema.

Shepherd's purse *Capsella bursa-pastoris*
Description: an annual or biennial with a basal rosette of pinnate leaves and branched stems and tiny white flowers appearing throughout the year. The plant produces characteristic heart-shaped seed pods, generally found on the stems alongside the flowers. It is a common garden weed growing to around 20 cm.
Parts used: aerial parts collected throughout the year
Actions: astringent, circulatory stimulant, diuretic, styptic, urinary antiseptic, uterine stimulant

Shepherd's purse takes its name from the heart-shaped seed pods which were thought to resemble the leather pouches once carried by shepherds. These same seed pods account for another of its country names – mother's hearts – and the plant (like others with "mother's…" or "lady's…" as part of their name) is a valuable gynaecological remedy helpful for menstrual irregularities and recommended as a tea in childbirth to encourage contractions and ease labour pains.

The herb can be eaten in salads, added to sandwiches and was once gathered and cooked as a spring vegetable: it has a pleasant, spicy flavour.

As well as having astringent and styptic properties, shepherd's purse is a urinary antiseptic and diuretic, so can be helpful in cystitis – it is especially suitable in severe cases where there is blood in the urine. Drinking the tea may help relieve heavy periods, while its astringency can also be helpful for chronic diarrhoea and in colitis.

The plant is also used in traditional Chinese medicine as an astringent styptic and wound healer, while the seeds are believed to help improve the eyesight. It has also been used to reduce fevers in malaria.

Caution: Shepherd's purse can cause contractions of the uterus, so should be avoided during pregnancy.

Cornflower *Centaurea cyanus*
Description: annual with grey-green lanceolate leaves and striking blue composite flowers in summer: some varieties have white or purple flowers.
Parts used: flowers collected when just open
Actions: astringent, anti-inflammatory, bitter, mild diuretic

The bright blue cornflower was once – like the red corn poppy – commonly found in summer cornfields across Europe. Increased use of agricultural chemicals has long since rid the farmer's acres of such attractive weeds and most cornflowers found today are in gardens or undisturbed wild areas.

In the Middle Ages the plant was known as bluebottle or blue bothem, but its wide use as a medicinal herb led to the adoption of the apothecaries' name – *flos frumenti* (which means literally "flower of the corn") – instead. Like its relative, centaury, cornflower contains a bitter compound (centaurine) which accounts for its use as a digestive stimulant. Cornflower tea made from the dried flowers is still used for indigestion in many parts of Europe and the bright blue flowers are often found in tisane mixtures in Austria and Hungary.

An infusion of the flowers is also a traditional folk remedy for tired eyes – use a cool, dilute, well-strained infusion in an eye-bath. Under the Doctrine of Signatures theory, cornflower was regarded as better for blue eyes; brown-eyed people were advised to use plantain instead. The flowers have a mild tonic effect. They make a useful and revitalising addition to early morning teas.

Greater celandine *Chelidonium majus*
Description: a perennial with brittle stems which yield a brilliant deep yellow sap. The leaves are divided with oblong leaflets, while the four-petalled flowers appear

Clockwise from top left: cornflower *Centaurea cyanus,* **greater celandine** *Chelidonium majus,* **hawthorn** *Crataegus oxycantha,* **hemp agrimony** *Eupatorium cannabinum*

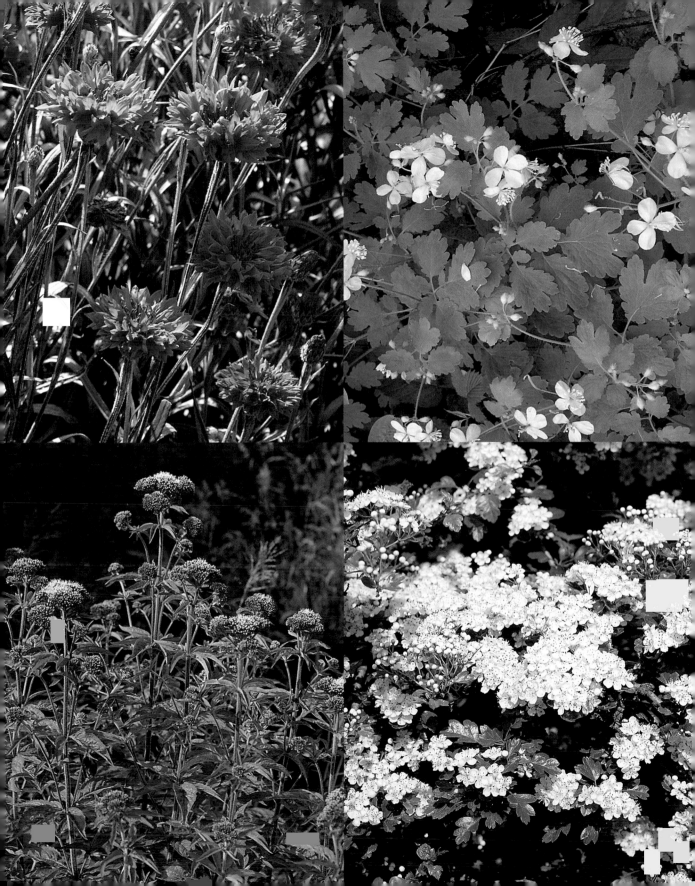

in summer and are followed by long, linear seed pods.

Parts used: aerial parts collected when flowering, sap

Actions: anti-inflammatory, antispasmodic, diuretic, bile stimulant, circulatory stimulant, laxative, uterine stimulant

Greater celandine is a member of the poppy family, completely unrelated to the lesser celandine or pilewort (see page 68), which belongs to the buttercup group. It is notable for its brilliantly coloured sap which makes an ideal remedy for clearing warts – simply apply a little each morning, taking care not to get too much of the juice on surrounding areas as it can be corrosive.

Internally the herb is used as a liver remedy, cleansing the gall bladder and stimulating bile flow in hepatitis and jaundice. It is also a diuretic and can be used as a cleansing remedy for skin conditions where liver stagnation is a contributing factor.

In the UK the use of greater celandine is restricted to professional practitioners only, although as the maximum dosage given in the legislation (200 ml of tincture per week) is at least three times what would normally be prescribed, it can be considered as safe and side-effect free in normal dosages.

An old name for the herb is "swallow wort", which dates from an ancient Greek tradition – repeated by herbalists as late as the 17th century – that swallows fed the seeds to their young to improve their eyesight. Certainly, the plant was widely recommended in the 17th century for eye complaints.

Caution: Excess can cause skin irritation, dry mouth, dizziness and drowsiness.

Hawthorn *Crataegus oxycantha*

Description: a common deciduous shrub or small tree, often used in hedging, with deeply lobed obovate leaves and pink or white scented flowers in late spring. Dark red oval fruits form in early autumn and are usually eaten by birds.

Parts used: flowering tops, collected in spring, and berries, collected when ripe in autumn

Actions: antispasmodic, astringent, heart tonic and restorative, normalises blood pressure, peripheral vasodilator, sedative

Like many members of the rose family, hawthorn is astringent and will help stop bleeding; as such it was largely used as a remedy for diarrhoea and heavy menstrual bleeding. Taking a Doctrine of Signatures approach, old herbals also recommend the plant for drawing thorns and splinters. It has been used for centuries as a hedging plant to divide farms and fields and the name "haw" is actually an old word for a hedge – hence hedgethorn.

Today we regard hawthorn primarily as a heart herb – a valuable tonic that will help normalise action and is widely used for high blood pressure. This is, however, a comparatively recent use as, apart from occasional mentions suggesting the herb as a remedy for dropsy (which can be related to blood pressure problems), there is little historic evidence linking hawthorn with heart disorders.

Now we know that it acts as a peripheral vasodilator, improving blood supply throughout the body as well as relaxing the coronary blood vessels, while it also has a general tonic effect on heart action and contains procyanadins which relax the central nervous system. It is used to reduce high blood pressure as well as counter the risk of angina attacks and helps to soften the fatty deposits of atherosclerosis which lead to hardening of the arteries. Both flowering tops and berries are used in this way, although the Chinese use only the berries and consider them primarily as a digestive remedy.

Hawthorn combined with linden flowers or yarrow makes a pleasant tea for those prone to high blood pressure. As an astringent, it is also worth remembering that hawthorn infusions can be used as a gargle for sore throats, a douche for vaginal discharges, and will be helpful for diarrhoea and other digestive upsets.

Rose-bay willow herb *Epilobium angustifolium*
Description: a tall, dramatic wild flower growing to 250 cm in height with brilliant pink flower spikes and long, narrow, minutely toothed leaves.
Parts used: aerial parts collected before and during flowering, root collected in autumn
Actions: some antibacterial action, astringent, demulcent, diuretic, styptic

In his classic book *The English Gardener*, William Cobbett, the 18th century writer, recommends rose-bay willow herb as an ideal plant to grow at the back of a shrubbery – its bright pink flowers well worth adding to the garden. Today we tend to condemn the plant to the "weed" category and eradicate it ruthlessly. It is certainly one of our more attractive wild flowers – Gerard called it a "goodly and stately plant".

Although little used in mainstream herbal medicine today, willow herb leaves were once dried and used as a substitute (and adulterant) for tea. Maud Grieve records that as late as the 1930s it was drunk regularly

in Russia as *kapoorie* tea. The young shoots were also boiled and eaten as a vegetable.

Medicinally, the root and leaves can be helpful for stomach upsets and gastroenteritis and can be ideal for diarrhoea in children. The root is made into a decoction using one teaspoon of chopped root to a cup of water, simmered for 15 minutes, and taken three times daily, while the leaves and flowers can be used in standard infusions (see page 25).

As an astringent rose-bay willow herb is useful as a gargle for sore throats and mouth ulcers; it was also once used in ointments for childhood eczema.

Hemp agrimony *Eupatorium cannabinum*
Description: A tall, sturdy plant with narrow leaves longer at the base and arranged in opposite pairs. The flowers form in dull pink clusters in late summer and early autumn.
Parts used: aerial parts, collected when flowering; roots collected in autumn
Actions: anti-scorbutic, bile stimulant, diuretic, expectorant, febrifuge, laxative, purgative and emetic in high doses, possible immune stimulant

An attractive wild plant generally found in damp places, hemp agrimony has been used since the days of Dioscorides as a laxative for constipation. It stimulates bile flow so can be helpful for liver stagnation and poor digestion. It was popular in the Middle Ages as a wound herb, and this may have been due to its anti-scorbutic action in countering the effects of scurvy.

Hemp agrimony is a useful remedy for colds and chills, helping to reduce fevers and ease coughs. Recent research suggests it may have antibiotic and immune-stimulating properties and it has also been found to contain a substance called eupatoriopicrin, which has anti-tumour properties.

As a diuretic and laxative, hemp agrimony can be useful for clearing toxins from the system in arthritis and chronic skin disorders. Poultices of the herb were once used on prurient skin sores.

The herb can be combined with elder flowers and yarrow to ease colds and chills, while a decoction of the root is a good expectorant for coughs and also has a laxative action. An infusion of the flowers and/or leaves can be helpful for rheumatic pains: when fresh the plant has rather more laxative active than when dried, so it needs to be used with caution.

Caution: High doses may cause nausea.

Meadowsweet *Filipendula ulmaria*
Description: a hardy perennial growing to around 120 cm in height and generally found in damp ditches and hedgerows. The plant has irregular pinnate leaves and large, fluffy, creamy flower heads which smell slightly of aspirin appearing from midsummer to early autumn.
Parts used: all the aerial parts, collected when flowering
Actions: mild analgesic, antacid, anti-inflammatory, anti-rheumatic, antiseptic, astringent, diaphoretic, diuretic, soothing for the gastric membranes

Meadowsweet's best known claim to fame is as the herb which gave us the name "aspirin". In the 1830s chemists first identified a substance called salicylic acid, extracted from willow bark, as an anti-inflammatory and analgesic, and over the following years worked to produce a synthetic drug. By the 1890s, the pharma-

ceutical company Bayer had finally patented the result and since salicylates extracted from meadowsweet had been involved in the development work, they named the drug aspirin after the old botanical name for meadowsweet, *Spiraea ulmaria*.

Crushed meadowsweet flowers certainly have an aspirin-like scent and the plant was used in Elizabethan times as a strewing herb to improve the smell of less than clean houses, as well as to flavour wine and ales. Meadowsweet has long been used in much the same way as the proprietary drug – for easing pains and feverish colds and as an anti-inflammatory for arthritic conditions.

Unlike aspirin, which can irritate the gastric lining and in prolonged use lead to ulceration, meadowsweet is extremely soothing and calming for the digestive tract. It is ideal for gastritis, indigestion and heartburn and is sometimes even described as having anti-ulcer activity. Meadowsweet infusion is excellent for many minor stomach upsets and taken after meals is good to counter indigestion: for digestive problems it combines well with marshmallow and lemon balm.

Strong extracts of meadowsweet are used by professional herbalists in treating arthritis and rheumatism, although in mild cases a home-made infusion can be useful. Increase the normal proportions to up to 60 g of dried herb to 500 ml of boiling water if need be.

Caution: Meadowsweet is best avoided by those sensitive to salicylates and aspirin.

Clockwise from top left: rose-bay willow herb *Epilobium angustifolium*, **meadowsweet** *Filipendula ulmaria*, **herb Robert** *Geranium robertianum*, **cleavers** *Galium aparine*

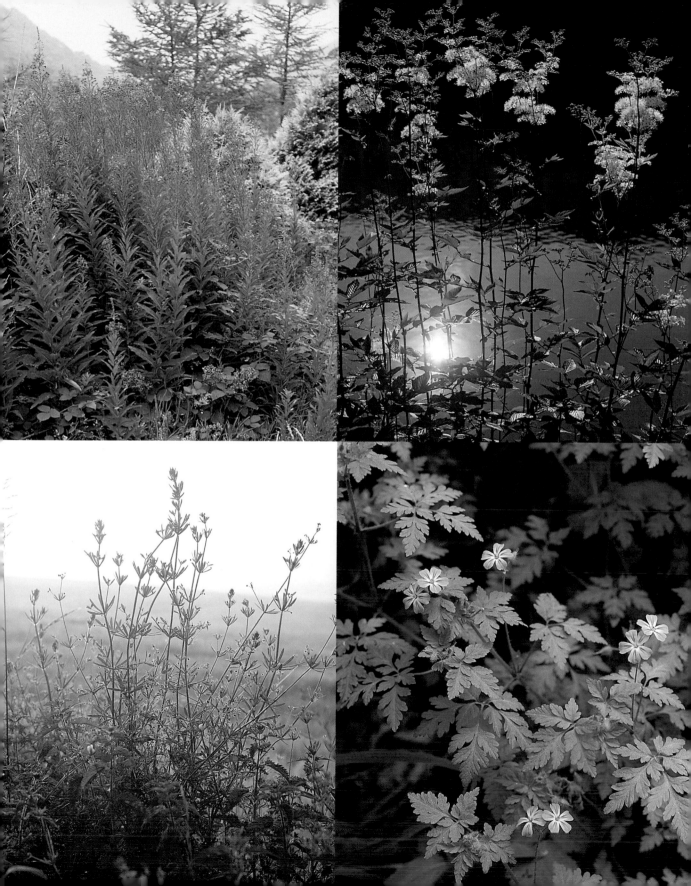

Cleavers *Galium aparine*

Description: a weedy, scrambling annual with whorls of up to nine elliptical leaves along the stem. Tiny green-white flowers appear beside these whorls in spring, followed by round purple-green fruits. The sticky stems will often spread for 3 m or more among shrubs and climbing plants.

Parts used: aerial parts, collected before fruiting

Actions: anti-inflammatory, astringent, diuretic, mild laxative, lymphatic cleanser

To most gardeners, cleavers – also known as sticky willy and sweetheart – is a pernicious weed with a fondness for scrambling through shrubs and threatening to choke prize specimens. Cleavers is also known as goosegrass and is a favourite food for these birds.

The herb is particularly valued for its tonic effect on the lymphatic system, making it a popular cleansing herb for skin problems and glandular disorders including tonsillitis, benign breast lumps, cysts, swollen lymph glands and glandular fever. It can also be made into creams and infused oils which will ease the symptoms of psoriasis.

The dried herb tends to display few diuretic properties (although it is popularly included in many over-the-counter products), but when used fresh as a juice it can be extremely effective and can be useful for both urinary disorders and fluid-retention problems associated with heart disease. Large amounts of the herb can easily be pulped in a food processor and drunk in wineglass doses three times a day.

The young shoots gathered in the spring also make a valuable seasonal cleansing tonic – eat them either fresh in salads and sandwiches, pulped or in teas.

Herb Robert *Geranium robertianum*

Description: an annual or biennial with red-tinged stems and highly divided, palmate leaves. The plant has a foetid smell and bright pink five-petalled flowers from early summer until mid to late autumn.

Parts used: whole plant (including the shallow roots), gathered during flowering

Actions: astringent, styptic, reduces blood sugar levels

All members of the geranium family are astringent, wound-healing and styptic and although the American cranesbill (*G. maculatum*) is most widely used in commercial herbalism, the British herb Robert is equally effective. It makes useful ground cover in the shrubbery, although it can easily become invasive. Its leaves have a slightly unpleasant, foetid smell when crushed – effective at keeping insects away, so rubbing exposed skin with the leaves can help prevent insect bites.

Herb Robert is believed to take its name from a medieval St Rupert and was once known as *herba sanctii ruperti* and widely used in folk medicine. Under Doctrine of Signatures theory, the plant's bright pink flowers and the reddish tinge to the stems suggested that it would be good for the blood and it was once used for haemorrhages and diabetes. Modern research does suggest it has some action in lowering blood sugar levels, although it is rarely used in this way today.

Herb Robert tea is suitably astringent to counter diarrhoea and the infusion can also be used as a gargle for mouth ulcers and sore throats or in an eye bath for conjunctivitis. The same infusion can also be used to bathe skin sores, minor cuts and grazes. Alternatively, the fresh leaves can be pounded to make a poultice for bruises and skin eruptions.

Wood avens *Geum urbanum*

Description: an upright perennial with slender stems and widely spaced pinnate leaves and small yellow flowers from early summer to mid-autumn. Purple-tinged fruits covered in hairy bristles appear in the autumn and the plant grows to around 60 cm. The root has a strong smell of cloves.

Parts used: aerial parts collected while flowering and roots dug in autumn

Actions: astringent, antiseptic, anti-inflammatory, digestive tonic, febrifuge, styptic

The plant is also known as herb Bennet or Benedict's herb a name derived from *herba benedicta* or blessed herb. In the Middle Ages its strong-smelling root was believed to ward off evil spirits and amulets of it were often worn or hung in homes to avert the evil eye. Although this belief in its potent effect on evil probably pre-dates Christianity, the plant is often seen in medieval illustration with the small trefoil-like stem leaves taken to symbolise the Trinity and the five-petalled flowers associated with the five wounds of Christ. The roots had symbolically to be collected on 25 March – Lady Day.

Its botanical name also focuses on this aromatic root: *geum* comes from a Greek word meaning "to produce a pleasant smell" – a smell which is easily lost when the root is dried, although fresh root can be used in cooking as an alternative to cloves.

Traditionally wood avens tea was taken for diarrhoea and to improve the appetite in debility and convalescence. Externally it has been used as a wound herb and gargling with the infusion – as with many astringent herbs – was once a folk remedy for sore throats and gum disease and can be useful as an anti-catarrhal.

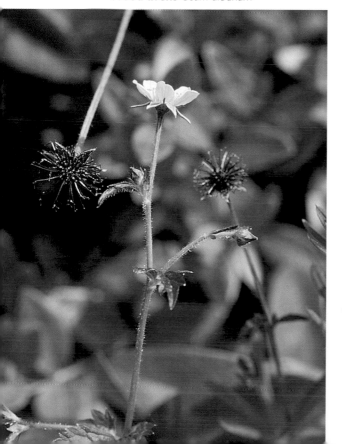

Wood avens *Geum urbanum*

St John's wort *Hypericum officinalis*

Description: an upright perennial growing from a woody base with linear ovate leaves which appear to be speckled with tiny holes when held to the light (they are, in fact, small oil sacs). The flowers are yellow with five petals and red-tipped stamens. It will grow to around 60 cm and flowers in midsummer.

Parts used: flowering tops collected in midsummer, leaves collected before or after flowering

Actions: astringent, analgesic, anti-inflammatory, anti-depressant, sedative, restorative tonic for the nervous system

St John's wort is believed to take its name from the Knights of St John of Jerusalem who used it as a wound herb on Crusade battlefields – although others suggest that it is associated with the midsummer rites of St John's Day (24 June) and the blood-red extracts that can be obtained from the herb. It is a good example of the Doctrine of Signatures, since the herb is helpful for inflammations and wounds.

The plant produces bright yellow flowers in early to midsummer and these can be collected and infused in sunflower oil for two weeks to produce a red oil which is ideal for soothing minor burns and sunburn.

St John's wort was believed to ward off evil spirits and the insane were often compelled to drink an infusion in an attempt to cure their madness. Today we know that the herb is an effective anti-depressant which is believed to inhibit the enzyme monoamine oxidase (MAO), which itself inhibits neurotransmitters involved in stimulating the brain. MAO inhibitors are widely used in orthodox medicine and some researchers suggest St John's wort has similar action but without the usual side effects of orthodox drugs.

It has become extremely popular in Germany where it is widely prescribed by general practitioners as a safe, effective and non-addictive alternative to tetracyclic drugs (a commonly prescribed group of orthodox anti-depresssants). Currently the herb is not licensed as an anti-depressant in the UK and several other countries, so over-the-counter products containing it can only claim to be a "sunshine herb" rather than a proven anti-depressant remedy.

The herb has long been regarded by herbalists as a restorative for the nervous system and it can ease pre-menstrual tension and some types of period pain. Recent interest has also focused on hypericins, found in the plant, which have an effect on the immune system and have been used in AIDS treatments.

Caution: Prolonged use may increase the photo-sensitivity of the skin.

White deadnettle *Lamium album*
Description: A hairy perennial with leaves reminiscent of the stinging nettle and square stems, characteristic of the mint family, to which it belongs. The white tubular, two-lipped flowers appear in whorls in the spring and early summer. The plant grows to around 60 cm in height.
Parts used: whole plant collected during flowering
Actions: anti-inflammatory, antispasmodic, astringent, diuretic, expectorant, menstrual regulator, styptic, vulnerary

White deadnettle – so called because its leaves resemble those of the stinging nettle, although it does not sting – is a common wild plant often growing as a weed in suburban gardens. It is no relation of the stinging nettle, but belongs to the mint family and takes its botanical name from the Greek word for throat, which was supposedly descriptive of the flowers.

These days the herb is mainly used for menstrual and urinary disorders: deadnettle tea can be helpful for cystitis and in prostatitis and it can speed recovery after

Clockwise from top left: St John's wort *Hypericum officinalis*, **white deadnettle** *Lamium album*, **toadflax** *Linaria vulgaris*, **purple loosestrife** *Lythrum salicaria*

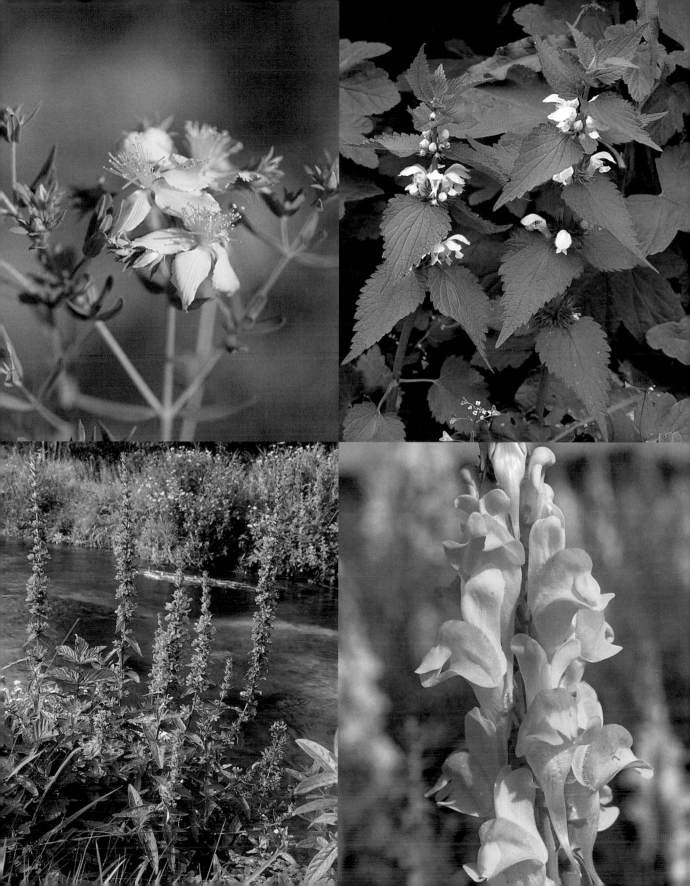

surgery for enlarged prostate. It can be taken for heavy periods and used as a douche for vaginal discharges.

White deadnettle also has some action on the bowel, helping to regulate function, so it can be useful for both constipation and diarrhoea. Externally, white deadnettle creams and ointments can be used on cuts and grazes and also make a soothing, astringent lotion for piles and burns.

The plant can also be eaten, with the young leaves and plant tips added to salads or cooked like spinach and served as a vegetable.

Toadflax *Linaria vulgaris*
Description: a slender perennial with thin, pointed leaves and yellow, snapdragon-like flowers in yellow and orange. It grows to around 90 cm and flowers throughout the summer.
Parts used: whole plant collected just before flowering
Actions: astringent, bitter, cleansing, diuretic, laxative, liver stimulant

Also known as "eggs and butter", the two-tone yellow flowers of toadflax not only provide the country name but were also seen as a "signature" for its therapeutic properties: yellow signified jaundice and in the 17th century the plant was widely used as a remedy for liver disorders. The leaves are rather like those of flax – hence the botanical name (from *linum* = flax) – while the "toad" part comes from a tradition that toads sheltered under its stems.

The plant has a cleansing effect on the liver and can still be used to treat hepatitis, gastroenteritis and gall bladder problems. Like many liver herbs, it has a role in treating skin disorders, including eczema and scrofula.

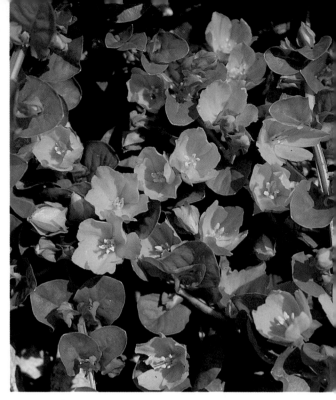

Creeping Jenny *Lysimachia nummularia*

Externally it can be used to bathe piles or made into a healing ointment for wounds, sores and skin rashes. The infusion was once recommended for eye inflammations. Drink toadflax tea as a cleansing remedy for the digestion or to stimulate the liver.

Creeping Jenny *Lysimachia nummularia*
Description: a creeping perennial usually found in damp meadows. Leaves are rounded on square stems with bright yellow cup-like flowers growing singly in the leaf axils in summer. A gold-leaved cultivar is often sold in garden centres.
Parts used: leaves, gathered before flowering
Actions: astringent, styptic, vulnerary

Once widely used as a wound herb, creeping Jenny is nowadays more likely to be found in an ornamental hanging basket than in the wild. The plant was originally found across Europe, from central Sweden to the Caucasus. In the garden it will meander happily through rockeries and around paving stones for 60 cm or more.

Its botanical name comes from the Latin *nummulus* for money and refers to the round, coin-like leaves – hence its alternative common name of moneywort. Ointment made from the fresh leaves was once a favourite for cuts and sores, while an infusion of the fresh leaves was taken for internal bleeding.

Gerard recommends the juice in wine for diarrhoea and blood in the stool, and adds that the plant boiled in wine with a little honey "prevaileth much against the cough in children" – a reference to its historic use as a specific for whooping cough. The leaves contain Vitamin C and were once taken, dried and powdered by Dutch sailors as a preventative for scurvy.

Purple loosestrife *Lythrum salicaria*
Description: a tall, upright perennial with bright purple flowers on whorled spikes from early summer to early autumn. The leaves resemble those of the willow and the plant will grow to around 150 cm in good growing conditions.
Parts used: aerial parts, gathered as they are coming into flower
Actions: anti-bacterial, astringent, diuretic, soothing, styptic

Usually found in damp, marshy areas, the tall flower spikes of purple loosestrife make an attractive addition to the late summer country lanes. The plant has been used medicinally since Roman times – Pliny talks of the smoke from burning loosestrife as driving away serpents and adds that the "power is so great that, if

placed on the yoke, when the beasts of burden are quarrelsome, it checks their bad temper".

The herb was once a popular European folk remedy for diarrhoea and dysentery and is still used like this in a number of over-the-counter products made in France and Switzerland. Research has shown that it can be effective against the amoeba which cause dysentery and can also combat the typhus bacilli.

Purple loosestrife makes a valuable wound herb – use the infusion as a wash to clean cuts and grazes. Internally it can be helpful for heavy periods or in severe cystitis where there is blood in the urine. It can be used to stop nosebleeds (apply a cotton wool swab soaked in the infusion or insert crushed leaves in the nostril). The tea can be used as a douche for vaginal discharges; or a strong decoction used externally as a wash on eczema, skin sores and ulcers. For diarrhoea use a decoction of the aerial parts rather than an infusion.

Common mallow *Malva sylvestris*
Description: a vigorous, hardy perennial with round, lobed leaves and purple, five-petalled flowers, appearing throughout the summer and autumn. The plant will grow to 120 cm.
Parts used: aerial parts collected during flowering
Actions: anti-bacterial, anti-tussive, demulcent, possible immune stimulant, mild laxative

Common mallow with its lobed leaves and bright purple flowers is a not unattractive common garden "weed" and hedgerow plant: it will, however, self-seed enthusiastically, so needs treating with caution in the garden. The botanical name derives from both the Latin *malva* and the Greek *malake*, which mean "soft" – a reference to its medical properties rather than to any particular softness of its leaves.

In the 16th century mallow was known as *omnimorbia* or cure-all and Gerard's list of its uses is certainly comprehensive, ranging from wasp stings to digestive upsets, tumours and the rather unpleasant sounding "inward burstings".

Mallow is closely related to both marshmallow and hollyhocks and all three have very similar medicinal properties: marshmallow (see page 120) is considered the strongest of the three and is the one normally chosen by medical herbalists, although common mallow makes a satisfactory alternative in an emergency.

The plant is rich in mucilage and is used as a soothing remedy for inflammations and irritation of the gastro-intestinal tract and also for coughs and bronchitis. The leaves and flowers are generally used; the root has similar actions but large doses can have a purgative effect. A poultice of mallow leaves is ideal for skin sores and inflammations.

Butterbur *Petasites hybridus*

Description: a dramatic plant growing to 200 cm with leaves up to 90 cm across and generally found in damp, marshy places. The flowers appear in early spring – before the leaves – in dense reddish spikes of either male or female blooms; they may be bell-shaped or thread-like and vary from pinks to purple.
Part used: roots collected in autumn
Actions: antispasmodic, astringent, diuretic, expectorant

Butterbur's botanical name comes from the Greek word *petatos*, which was the term for a shepherd's felt hat and is descriptive of the large, soft leaves: butterbur

leaves and stems make a useful parasol for sunny days. In the past the leaves were used to wrap butter – hence the common name.

Butterbur is a popular medicinal herb in mainland Europe and extracts are found in many Swiss and German over-the-counter products, although there are some concerns about its toxicity as it contains traces of pyrrolizidine alkaloids (see Comfrey, page 142).

The herb was traditionally used in European folk medicine as a cough remedy, while Gerard recommended it for the plague: "…because it provoketh sweat and driveth from the harte all venome and ill heat" and suggested that it "killeth wormes". He also urged the use of butterbur in ale for "pestilent and burning fevers".

While these traditional applications of butterbur have largely fallen into disuse recent research has demonstrated that the plant has considerable anti-spasmodic and pain-relieving properties, making it suitable for tension headaches, migraine and period pain. Other researchers have shown that it can affect digestive function and is helpful for gastritis, gall bladder spasms and stomach upsets. The root, flowers and leaves have all been used medicinally in the past, although the root is generally regarded as the most efficacious and a decoction is ideal for home use.

It is best to collect butterbur from the wild rather than attempting to cultivate it in the garden: nothing will grow under its vast leaves and it can spread rapidly and prove very difficult to eradicate.

Clockwise from top left: butterbur *Petasites hybridus,* **self-heal** *Prunella vulgaris,* **ribwort plantain** *Plantago lanceolata,* **comon mallow** *Malva sylvestris*

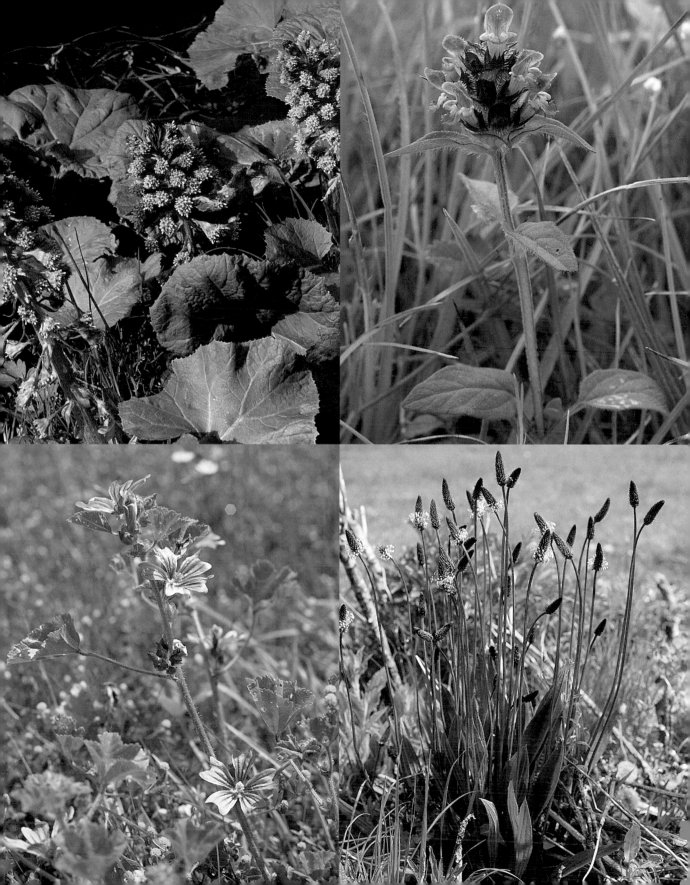

Plantain *Plantago* spp.

Description: common plantain (*P. major*) is characterised by its rat tail-like flower spikes and basal rosette of fleshy, rounded or ovate leaves. It grows to around 15 cm high and is commonly found in gardens and pavement cracks. Ribwort plantain (*P. lanceolata*) is taller, up to 75 cm, with more pointed, lance-shaped leaves with three to five prominent ribs. Its flowers are dark rust with clear white feathery stamens and appear from late spring to early autumn.

Part used: leaves

Actions: common plantain – anti-bacterial, anti-histamine, anti-allergenic, astringent, blood tonic, demulcent, diuretic, expectorant, styptic; ribwort plantain – anti-catarrhal, antispasmodic, relaxing expectorant, tonifies mucous membranes

Common plantain was known as "white man's foot" in North America as the native tribes watched it spread with the settlers. The plant is a familiar garden weed, often found filling the cracks in crazy paving and dominating lawns. To the Anglo-Saxons it was "waybread" – one of the nine sacred herbs given to mankind by Woden and listed in the ninth-century poem the *Lacnunga*. The plant has long been regarded as an important healing herb – Pliny even suggests that if several pieces of flesh are put in a pot with plantain they will join back together again.

Externally the leaves are a good emergency treatment for irritant insect bites, while internally common plantain tea – made from the leaves – can be helpful for gastric irritations, irritable bowel, piles, cystitis or heavy periods. Plantain juice, mixed with honey, is a soothing remedy for cuts and minor wounds.

Common plantain's close relative, ribwort, is more likely to be found in the wild. It is used for colds, hay fever and allergic rhinitis, but also contains minerals and trace elements – particularly zinc, potassium and silica – so can act as a tissue healer and immune stimulant. The presence of aucubin, an antibiotic chemical, helps to make it healing and supportive for the immune system.

Self-heal *Prunella vulgaris*

Description: an invasive, creeping perennial commonly found as a garden weed and one that readily invades lawns. It has oblong ovate leaves and deep-purple, lipped flowers produced in compact spikes which ripen to produce brown spiked seed pods in autumn.

Parts used: whole plant collected during flowering, flower heads collected in midsummer

Actions: alterative, anti-bacterial, astringent, bitter, cooling, diuretic, hypotensive, tonifies liver and gall bladder, vulnerary

As its common name implies, self-heal is a well-established European wound herb, widely used to stop bleeding from "inward and outward wounds". The flower spikes were considered to resemble the throat and under the Doctrine of Signatures theory, it was also used for inflammations of the mouth and throat. In fact the botanical name, *Prunella* – or so William Cole argued in 1657 – is derived from a German word *die Breuen*, meaning mouth.

Self-heal can be useful for all sorts of bleeding – including heavy periods where there is no known cause, and blood in the urine from severe cystitis.

Top: elder *Sambucus nigra;*
bottom: yellow dock *Rumex crispus*

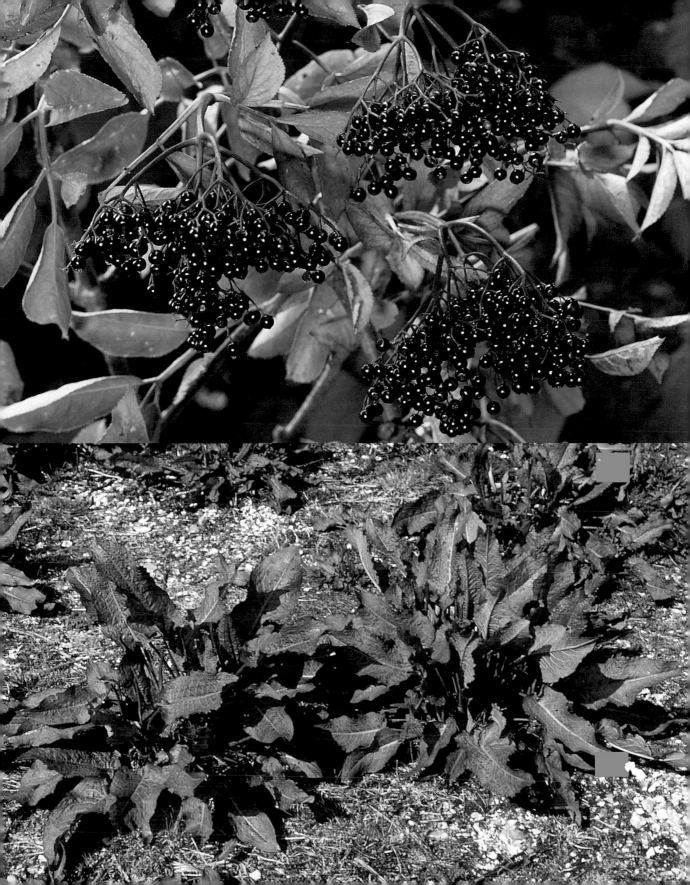

The same plant is used in Chinese medicine where it is known as *Xia Ku Cao* – which literally means "summer dry herb". In China only the flower spikes are used and are considered especially cooling for the liver. The herb is prescribed for any condition associated with what the Chinese term "liver fire" and generally characterised by irritability, anger, headaches and high blood pressure. The same remedy can also help calm hyperactive children – take it as an infusion up to four times a day.

Use an infusion of the whole herb as a wash for cuts and grazes or apply crushed, washed whole leaves as a poultice.

Yellow dock *Rumex crispus*

Description: a biennial growing to around 150 cm in height with a robust tap root and long-stalked ovate leaves up to 50 cm in length. The flowers are purple and thistle-like, appearing from early summer to mid-autumn and followed by hooked fruits.

Part used: root

Actions: alterative, bitter tonic, bile stimulant, laxative

Yellow dock is generally found growing in wild, grassy places, waste land and along the road side. The plant is able to concentrate iron from the soil in its roots thus making a valuable iron tonic in anaemia: in the past herbalists sprinkled iron filings around their yellow dock plants to produce iron-enriched specimens.

Yellow dock is mainly used as a cleansing remedy for skin and rheumatic problems. It contains anthraquinone glycosides which encourage peristalsis by irritating the gut lining, so have a purging effect; the plant is also useful for stimulating liver function and for itching skin conditions and shingles.

In Galenical medicine, yellow dock was considered as sufficiently cooling to purge the "choleric" humour or yellow bile. Culpeper considered it more effective than its close relatives sorrel and red dock and also recommended the seeds – no longer commonly used in herbal medicine – as a remedy for diarrhoea and stomach upsets. In homoeopathy, yellow dock extracts are used in cough mixtures and to relieve irritated sore throats.

Use the root in decoctions for rheumatic pains and digestive complaints.

Elder *Sambucus nigra*

Description: a large shrubby tree with pinnate leaves and tiny, scented cream flowers borne in flat bunches in early summer. The purple berries ripen in late autumn.

Parts used: flowers collected in spring and berries in autumn; the bark, leaves and root have all been used in the past – collect the leaves in summer after flowering.

Actions: anti-inflammatory, anti-catarrhal, diaphoretic, diuretic, emollient (flowers), laxative (berries and bark)

In the Middle Ages, many people believed that the elder tree was inhabited by a spirit known as the "elder mother" whose permission was needed if ever the tree was to be pruned; inevitably felling elders was considered as a guarantee of bad luck, although branches from the tree placed over doors and windows were believed to keep witches away and ward off the Evil Eye. According to Maud Grieve, author of the well-known *Modern Herbal* (1931), country people in the 1920s would still doff their hats when passing an elder tree as a salute to this otherwise forgotten sprite.

Such respect was understandable, since the elder was a complete medicine chest. The leaves formed the basis of a "green ointment" for sprains and strains, the inner bark is a strong purgative, the berries – a good source of Vitamin C – protected against colds and infections, while the flowers are strongly anti-catarrhal.

Today we mainly use the flowers as a soothing anti-catarrhal and diaphoretic remedy, although they are also topically anti-inflammatory and emollient and make a very effective hand cream: elder flower water (from distilling the flowers) was a favourite in the 18th century for whitening the skin and removing freckles.

Elder flowers also appear to strengthen the mucous membranes, so can increase resistance to irritant allergens. Drinking elder flower tea in early spring can help reduce hay fever symptoms later in the year. An infused oil of elder leaves also makes a useful alternative to the old "green ointment" to treat bruises and minor injuries.

Marsh woundwort *Stachys palustris*

Description: hardy perennial with tuberous roots and hairy, lanceolate leaves. It has dark red or purple flowers in summer borne on tall spikes flowering from the base. It has an unpleasant smell when crushed.
Parts used: aerial parts, collected while flowering
Actions: antiseptic, antispasmodic, astringent, styptic, tissue healer

Country names often provide a clue to a plant's healing action and marsh woundwort is no exception. Gerard called it "clown's woundwort" with the "clown" suggesting that the herb was widely used by the common people.

The leaves of marsh woundwort were once pounded with animal fats to make an ointment for fresh wounds which was deemed so effective that the injury would "heale in such short time and in such absolute manner that it is hard for any that hath not the experience thereof to believe". Gerard was a great enthusiast for the plant and his *Herball* details how he cured one Edmund Cartwright who had been badly injured in a duel – "thrust through the thorax" – with an ointment of marsh woundwort and a little rose oil.

The herb grows in damp places but will thrive in most suburban gardens. As well as its healing actions, marsh woundwort is antispasmodic and taken as a tea can be helpful for cramp. Folk tradition also suggests the aerial parts as a remedy for gout and vertigo.

Chickweed *Stellaria media*

Description: a common annual weed forming low-growing mats of slender stems with oval leaves and small, white, star-like flowers appearing from early spring to early autumn.

Chickweed *Stellaria media* (greatly enlarged)

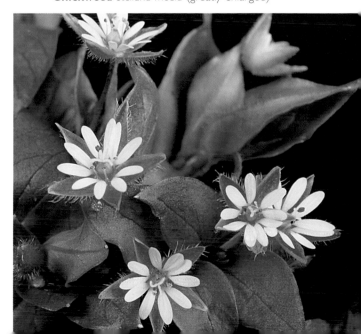

Parts used: aerial parts, gathered throughout the year whenever the plant appears
Actions: alterative, anti-rheumatic, cooling, demulcent, mild laxative, vulnerary, counters itching

Chickweed, as the name suggests, is a favourite food for domestic fowl. In Elizabethan times it was fed to caged birds and in the Middle Ages was known as *morsus gallinae* or hen's bite. It is a common garden weed, once gathered as a vegetable to be cooked like spinach and tossed in butter or else used as a salad herb.

Soothing and astringent, chickweed's main medicinal use is in creams and ointments for irritant skin rashes and eczema, or in the first-aid box for burns, boils and drawing splinters. Culpeper suggests combining chickweed with rose petals and adding various pig and sheep fats to create an extremely soothing ointment – it would certainly be a good combination, as rose petals have long been regarded as supportive for "the skin and the soul". The whole flowering chickweed plant can be made into infused oils (using the hot method described on page 32) and added to bath water to soothe skin problems. Use 10 ml of the infused oil in a warm bath.

Chickweed poultices were once a favourite for rheumatic pains, gout and also varicose ulcers.

Although not so popular as an internal remedy it is particularly cooling and can be worth adding to mixtures for rheumatism and hot, irritant skin conditions. The leaves are a useful source of Vitamin C.

Comfrey *Symphytum officinale*
Description: a robust, erect (up to 120 cm) perennial with thick, mucilaginous roots and large, ovate leaves.

The funnel-shaped flowers appear in clusters in summer and can be white to purple.
Parts used: root, collected in autumn, or leaves, collected during early flowering
Actions: astringent, demulcent, expectorant, tissue healer, cell proliferant

Although comfrey has been used for centuries as a wound healer and restorer of broken bones – its country name is "knitbone" and the botanical name is derived from the Greek *sympho* meaning to unite – it has had a more chequered history in recent years, veering from panacea to health hazard.

Its healing action is due to a chemical called allantoin which encourages growth of various tissue cells and so accelerates healing. Generations used comfrey poultices on pulled ligaments and minor fractures, while herbalists used it internally for stomach ulceration. The immense healing properties of the plant have been put to many diverse uses over the centuries: in the past comfrey baths were popular before marriage in the belief that they would repair the hymen and thus create the appearance of virginity.

During the 1960s and 1970s the plant became over-hyped as a cure-all for arthritis and this inevitably focused research interest on its constituents. Scientists fed large amounts of the plant to rats which subsequently died of liver disease and comfrey's pyrrolizidine alkaloids were blamed. Comfrey supporters argue that the rats had so much comfrey to eat they actually suffered from the effects of malnutrition and maintain that the alkaloids are not extracted in conventional

Dandelion *Taraxacum officinale*

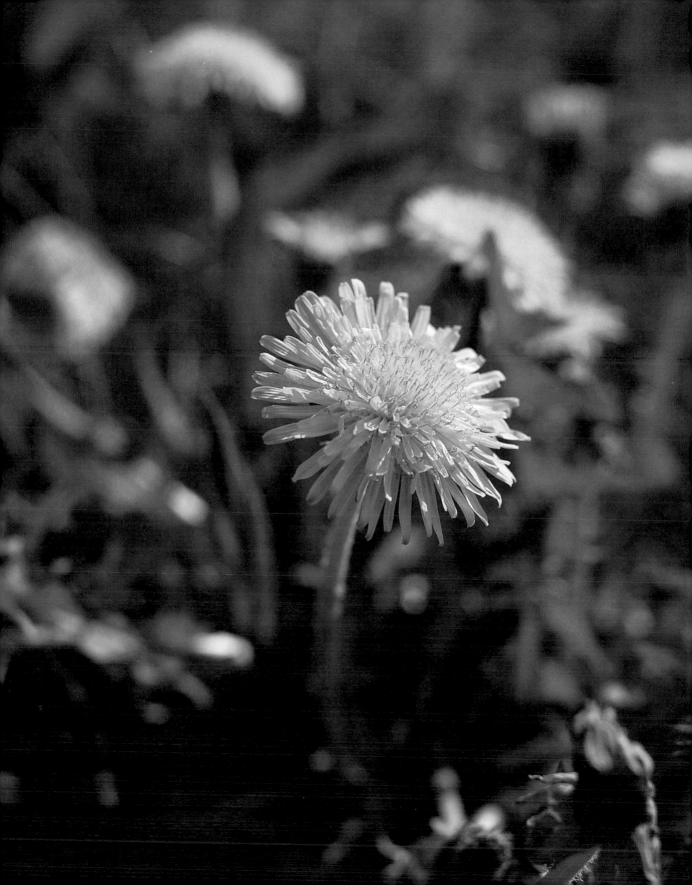

herbal preparations (infusions and ointments). Health authorities have tended to disagree and comfrey is now banned in many parts of the world, including Australia. In the UK the leaf can still be sold over-the-counter and it can be used in external preparations, although many advise against using it on open wounds.

The herb is still easily found in the wild or can be grown in gardens (although it does have tenacious roots). The hot infused oil is easy to make and forms a useful base for massage oils for arthritis, sprains and similar traumatic injuries – add 2-5 drops of rosemary or lavender essential oil to 10 ml of comfrey, and rub into aching joints and limbs. Regular treatment can help repair the damage of old injuries which may be contributing to osteoarthritis. Comfrey is also extremely healing for any sort of bruising.

The dangers of pyrrolizidine alkaloids apart, the herb should not be used on fresh wounds before they are thoroughly cleaned since the rapid healing caused by the allantoin may trap dirt, so leading to abscesses.

Dandelion *Taraxacum officinale*
Description: perennial with a long tap root and a basal rosette of toothed leaves. Erect yellow composite flowers appear from spring to autumn followed by the characteristic puffball of hairy seeds.
Parts used: root generally gathered in spring, leaves gathered before flowering
Actions: anti-rheumatic, bile stimulant, diuretic, mild laxative, liver and digestive tonic

Use of dandelion in Western medicine is first mentioned in the *Ortus Sanitatis* of 1485, making it a comparative newcomer to the repertoire. The name

dandelion was apparently invented by a 15th-century surgeon known only as Master Wilhelm, who compared the shape of the leaves to a lion's tooth or *dens leonis*. Initially the herb was regarded as a variant of endive or chicory and recommended as a liver remedy. Its botanical name actually derives from the Arabic *tarakhaqún*, which means "wild chicory". The leaves are still eaten in salad (especially in France) and have a noted diuretic action – hence the French name, *pissenlit*, and Old English *pissabed* or *piddlybeds*.

Master Wilhelm and his contemporaries regarded dandelion as a cooling herb, as do the Chinese. They have used it in medicine since the seventh century and recommend it for both liver problems and skin eruptions, where it is considered to "cool the blood".

As a diuretic, dandelion is unusual in that it is extremely rich in potassium, which is generally lost in urination. Although the whole plant has a tonic action on the liver, the root is rather more stimulating and cleansing and dandelion root tea makes a good laxative and liver stimulant for a sluggish digestion.

The plant is also anti-inflammatory and useful as a cleansing remedy in rheumatism, although it is mainly included in remedies for kidney and liver problems.

It is commonly included in over-the-counter slimming preparations for its diuretic and laxative properties – although this is not an ideal way to attempt to lose weight, as it simply depletes body fluids.

Dandelion leaves are very nutritious (rich in Vitamins A, B-complex, and C, plus iron, manganese, phosphorus, sulphur, manganese, calcium, silica and potassium), so are

Clockwise from top left: marsh woundwort *Stachys palustris,* **comfrey** *Symphytum officinale,* **stinging nettle** *Urtica dioica,* **coltsfoot** *Tussilago farfara*

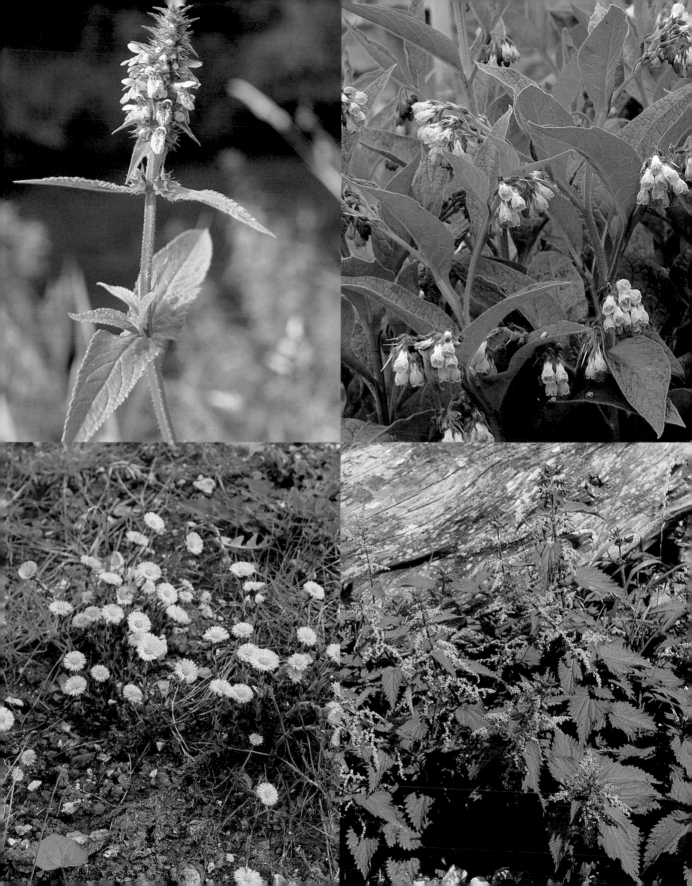

well worth adding to salads. Dandelion leaf tea can help with mild fluid retention and a decoction of the root makes a cleansing drink for the liver. Dandelion is unusual in that it is generally recommended to gather the roots in the spring rather than autumn, when most roots are lifted. This is because the starch content is lower then, so the active medicinal constituents are in greater concentration. However, the French recommend the juice of the root, gathered in autumn, as a liver tonic.

Externally the white sap from dandelion stems can be used on warts, while an infusion of aerial parts has been used for in an eye-bath for eye inflammations.

Coltsfoot *Tussilago farfara*

Description: a creeping perennial with round or heart-shaped leaves with a cobweb-like surface pattern. The flowers look rather like short, tufted dandelions on scaly stems and appear before the leaves in early spring.

Parts used: flowers collected in spring, leaves collected in summer

Actions: anti-catarrhal, antispasmodic, anti-inflammatory, anti-tussive, demulcent, relaxing expectorant, diuretic

Coltsfoot was once one of our most popular remedies for coughs and catarrh – its botanical name comes from the Latin for "cough dispeller" – however, its use has declined in recent years and, indeed, has been banned in some countries due to the discovery of pyrrolizidine alkaloids in the leaves. These chemicals are known, in extremely high doses, to cause liver disease in rats (see pages 142–144), although there is no firm evidence to suggest that coltsfoot can cause similar damage. Even

so, it has fallen from favour and many herbalists advise its short-term use only.

The plant is unusual in that its flowers appear (in early spring) before the leaves, hence its old name *filius ante patrem*, meaning the son before the father. The flowers can be difficult to find so it is always best to identify your coltsfoot patch during the preceding summer when you gather leaves and then return in spring to collect the flowers. It is a virulent weed and can be very difficult to eradicate from gardens, so is best gathered from the wild.

The yellow flowers can be dried or made into syrups; the leaves can be collected later in the year and similarly processed. Flowers and leaves (or the relevant syrups) are both used in the West, and can be combined as desired, although in traditional Chinese medicine only the flowers are used (also for coughs and catarrh). Coltsfoot is an extremely effective soothing expectorant and anti-catarrhal, especially helpful for irritating and spasmodic coughs, including whooping cough, asthma and bronchitis.

Stinging nettle *Urtica dioica*

Description: a coarse perennial with ovate, toothed leaves covered with hairs. The flowers are small and green and hang in drooping clusters up to 10 cm long. The plant has creeping yellow roots and can be difficult to eradicate.

Parts used: aerial parts, roots, gathered before flowering

Actions: antiseptic, anti-rheumatic, astringent, blood tonic, diuretic, expectorant, galactagogue, hypotensive, lowers blood sugar levels, important source of minerals, clears uric acid

Stinging nettles were once used in a rather bizarre treatment known as urtication which involved beating paralysed limbs with the plant in an attempt to stimulate sensations. The same remedy was also recommended for rheumatic pains, while the Romans reputedly planted the small annual continental nettle (*U. pilulifera*) along British roads because they believed the country was so cold they would need to beat their bodies with nettles to keep warm.

Nettles sting because the hairs on their stems and leaves contain histamine, which is a potent skin irritant. Thanks to their ability to "rob the soil" and concentrate minerals and vitamins in their leaves they are a good nutrient and the plant makes a useful "spring tonic" as well as a good supplement in iron-deficient anaemia.

Processing fresh young nettles in a juicer is a good way to make an energising tonic; they can also be cooked in soups to help clear out the stagnations of winter.

Nettles can be used externally in washes or infused oils for irritant skin rashes and the same oil can be used as the base for a massage rub for rheumatism. Internally, nettle tea is a popular folk remedy for rheumatism and can also help to relieve the acute painful stage of gout. In pregnancy, nettle tea makes a useful additional source of calcium and iron and it also stimulates milk flow when breast-feeding. Drinking nettle tea can be helpful for allergic skin rashes, especially those connected with salicylate sensitivity (see page 172). The plant will also reduce blood sugar levels, so is a useful addition to dietary control of late-onset diabetes.

Part 3: Using herbs for common ailments

In an ideal world we would always have the right herb available whenever we need it: the creams ready to cope with sudden sprains, the cough mixture sitting waiting for the first sign of a tickle. Few of us are that organised – even professional herbalists occasionally find themselves out of stock of a remedy just when it is needed. At times we all have to substitute alternative herbs or combinations of herbs which will perform the same task adequately. It is then that we begin to appreciate the real versatility of some plants: one could almost list 101 uses for the humble cabbage which can be applied to all manner of ills and the same is true of onion, ginger, St John's wort and marigold.

For home use herbal choice is limited as much by such practicalities as the size of the bathroom cabinet as by what happens to be available from local health food shops or in the wild. Personal preferences also play a part: some would be happy to rub garlic on their acne pustules; others will refuse even to eat such an aromatic plant.

The healing plants covered in Part 2 were chosen as being readily available from high street shops or – in the main – specimens that are commonly found in gardens or the countryside.

In this section ailments are grouped by bodily system with a list of key herbs that are especially suitable for those categories of ailments, as well as individual suggestions. If you do not have the recommended plant available, check the information given for the key herbs in Part 2 to find a suitable substitute.

Aches and *pains*

No matter how healthy their lifestyles sooner or later most people have some experience of muscular aches and pains: it could be a pulled muscle or ligament due to accidental injury, the wear and tear of osteoarthritis or even that new ill of the 20th century, repetitive strain injury. Or it could be a less localised problem – a systemic disorder such as rheumatoid arthritis or, more commonly, a nagging backache which seems to have no obvious cause.

Orthodox treatment usually focuses on "painkillers", but pain is only a symptom, there to remind us that the body is out of balance and in need of rest and repair. Sometimes the pain and the cause are closely associated – slipped discs cause back pain, fractured wrists hurt – but it is not always the case. In traditional Chinese medicine five-element theory (see page 9) the liver is associated with the tendons, the kidney with the bones, and the muscles or flesh with the spleen. Unexplained joint or muscle problems can therefore suggest a primary weakness in one or other of these organs. This is often seen with knee pain and liver disharmony. The knees contain rather a lot of tendons, so if these tissues are showing signs of weakness, the knees can be the first joints affected. A typical result of liver abuse – in the form of too much alcohol or rich food – can often be aching knees the next morning.

The same applies to those vague backaches: often they can be related to energy imbalances elsewhere in the body and can be significant signs of these disorders. Kidney weakness, for example, can be accompanied by low-back pain or

the ache could be related to a gynaecological problem.

The sorts of aches and pains that respond well to home remedies include sprains, strains, traumatic injuries including bruises, and those occasional twinges caused by old injuries – usually when the weather changes – that can lead to osteoarthritis in later life: all the sort of ailments, in fact, that the orthodox first-aider would treat with aspirin or painkilling sprays.

First choice in herbal remedies often lies with the essential oils. These are the "magic bullets" of the herbal repertoire: quick-acting, entering the blood stream almost immediately when applied to the skin, and – having bypassed the liver – quickly unleashing potent chemicals into the circulation. Essential oils are expensive and can be subject to adulteration by the unscrupulous, with synthetic chemicals added on a massive and hazardous scale. For home use choose branded products offering some sort of quality guarantee and always dilute in a carrying medium, such as sweet almond oil or water, before use (see page 34).

Sprains and pulled muscles

Pulled muscles and twisted joints can be acutely painful and if they result from some accidental, traumatic injury, an X-ray is often necessary to identify fractures or cracked bones. Strains involve a slight tearing of a muscle or the tendon attaching it to a bone and are generally caused by over-stretching. Sprains are a tear in the joint capsule or associated ligaments caused by twisting.

Comfrey and arnica are ideal for treating any damaged tissue: apply a little cream, ointment or infused oil and rest

the injured area as much as possible. Arnica can be particularly useful for relieving pain, while comfrey increases cell growth and so speeds healing. Avoid using both ointments if the skin is broken: arnica can be irritant, while comfrey is under suspicion for containing toxic alkaloids (see page 142) and it can also speed healing to such an extent that dirt may be trapped in cuts and grazes leading to abscesses.

Twisted or strained muscles often respond well to herbal rubs. Massage oils containing eucalyptus, lavender, thyme or rosemary can also be effective.

For accidental sprains and pulled muscles a useful massage oil can be made from 10 drops each of essential oils of rosemary and lavender with 5 drops each of essential oil of thyme and eucalyptus, all in 20 ml of good quality carrier oil, such as sweet almond or wheatgerm oil, or infused comfrey oil. Massage the mixture gently and frequently into the affected area for 24-36 hours to provide pain relief and encourage repair.

A useful alternative is simply to apply a cabbage poultice – crush a leaf with a vegetable mallet and wrap it around the injured limb, securing with a loose bandage. Fresh comfrey leaf, crushed daisies or hot mashed potato can be used in the same way.

Backache

Backache is one of our most common ailments: causes can range from pulled muscles and damaged discs (the spongy plugs that separate the vertebrae and act as shock absorbers) to poor posture, kidney disease, gynaecological problems or simply sitting in an awkward position for long periods.

Some sorts of backache are dignified by rather grander names: "lumbago" simply means pain in the lower back (the lumbar region) from whatever cause, whereas "sciatica" is a pain felt along the back and outer side of the thigh, leg and foot, with accompanying back pain and stiffness, often caused by a damaged disc putting pressure on the sciatic nerve. "Fibrositis" is an inflammation of fibrous tissue, especially muscle sheaths, which often affects the back muscles. It leads to pain and stiffness and can be treated with anti-inflammatories and those remedies recommended for rheumatic disorders (see below).

All these various sorts of backache require very different treatment, so accurate diagnosis is important if therapy is to be at all relevant. If the problem originates from mechanical damage in the back itself, treatment from an osteopath or chiropractor can often solve the problem; massage from a remedial masseur or physiotherapist can also give relief, while poor posture can be helped by learning the Alexander Technique through a series of lessons.

For persistent backache with no obvious cause, changing sleeping arrangements can sometimes help: mattresses should give support (they don't have to be hard!) and putting an extra pillow under the mattress to raise the top of the bed can be worth trying. It can also be useful to alternate lying on your back with knees bent and then curling into a small ball with the spine curved, as in the foetal position, as you fall off to sleep.

As well as using massage oils containing juniper, rosemary, lavender, thyme or eucalyptus, add 2-3 drops of these same essential oils to a hot bath.

For backache related to kidney weakness, drinking buchu and cinnamon tea can be helpful: use one teaspoon of buchu leaves and a generous pinch of dried cinnamon to a cup of boiling water and infuse for 10 minutes. Repeat up to three times a day for up to a week.

Rheumatism and arthritis

Rheumatism is a very imprecise term used to describe various chronic muscular aches and pains. It can include fibrositis and lumbago and may be referred to as "myalgia", which just means pain in the muscles. Arthritis simply means an inflammation of a joint, although as there are various types of arthritis requiring rather different treatment it is important to be sure of the exact diagnosis.

Osteoarthritis is generally due to "wear and tear" – youthful injuries to joints that have never fully healed or obesity putting excessive strain on the weight-bearing joints. Typically in osteoarthritis the protective cartilage surrounding the bones of a joint becomes damaged and wears away, causing the bones to rub together and become deformed. Joints often creak, become stiff and painful, while movement is often limited.

Rheumatoid arthritis (RA) is a more serious and potentially crippling disease that always requires professional treatment. It is an inflammatory problem and may be hereditary. The cause is often unknown but it affects joints symmetrically, commonly attacking both hands, both knees or both sides of the jaw. Inflammation leads to destruction of cartilage and eventually bone, with severe bone deformity.

Arthritis can also occur in children and may be of the inflammatory rheumatoid variety or a more complex syndrome. Juvenile arthritis also needs professional medical treatment.

Chronic arthritis may be related to food intolerance and eliminating possible allergens – especially dairy products, wheat, gluten, beef or pork – can prove extremely helpful. Many arthritics also find that refined carbohydrates (e.g. products made from white sugar and white flour), citrus fruits, tomatoes and excessive amounts of red meat increase symptoms, while recent research suggests that generally reducing animal fats in the diet can bring relief.

There is also some evidence that arthritic problems of sudden onset could be triggered by a bacterial infection or possibly a virus, so it can be worth adding echinacea, garlic or shiitake mushrooms to the diet to help the immune system.

Localised osteoarthritic problems can respond to topical, long-term treatment. Comfrey, for example, helps to repair the damage from old injuries and rubbing a little comfrey cream into the joint each night can, over a period of many months, bring relief.

As an alternative to the orthodox painkillers and anti-inflammatories, try hot herbal massage oils and poultices. Essential oil of rosemary (10 drops to 10 ml of carrier oil) makes an ideal lotion for "rheumatic" twinges. If used as soon as symptoms appear, it can generally stop those nagging aches developing to the stage when painkillers would usually be needed. Equally effective are hot infused oils made from chili, ginger, horseradish and pepper (or a combination of all of them), which will encourage blood flow to the area and warm cold joints. These oils should be used in moderation as they can cause skin blistering in some people.

Longer-term herbal treatment usually involves the use of cleansing herbs to remove any chemical toxins lingering in the tissues. Diuretics, digestive stimulants, circulatory stimulants and laxatives can all be helpful in treating chronic conditions. Relevant plants include birch, borage, burdock, celery, cucumber, grapes, meadowsweet, pears, pineapples, rosemary, watercress and yellow dock, which can be added to the menu or taken in teas. Anti-inflammatories, such as devil's claw, can also help, while many people successfully use feverfew for arthritis, although it can have side effects (see page 72).

There are also suggestions that congenital rheumatic conditions (especially RA) may be due to the body's inability to manufacture *gamma*-linolenic acid (see page 184), so supplements of evening primrose or borage oil can be worth trying. Extra calcium may also be helpful, especially among post-menopausal women.

In Ayurvedic medicine, joint pain is a characteristic of *vata* – air or wind – and arthritis is termed *amavata* or toxic air. It is associated with injury or with weak digestive fire leading to a build-up of toxins which are eventually carried to the joints. Arthritis can be further classified by the three Ayurvedic humours (air, water and fire): the *pitta* or fire type is what we would term rheumatoid arthritis, where the pain is relieved by cold compresses rather than rubefacients; *kapha*-type involves more joint swelling and oedema and is worse in damp weather; while

vata-type is more cold and dry in character. The cold-damp variety (the sort most likely to be seen in a cold, damp climate) is treated much as Galen would have recommended with hot, dry herbs like mustard and ginger, while patients are recommended to avoid damp and heavy foods – a category which in Ayurveda includes meats, cereals, nuts and milk.

In traditional Chinese medicine, arthritic or rheumatic aches and pains are termed *Bi* syndrome and are blamed on attack by external evils. These evils may have been successful because the energy protecting the body – the *Wei Qi* – is weak (hence the usefulness of immune-stimulants and anti-bacterials in therapy). Several variants of *Bi* can be identified, including "wind" (hence the shifting nature of the arthritic twinges afflicting different joints at different times), "cold and damp", which is comparable to osteoarthritis with joint swellings, and "hot *Bi*", which is a more apt description of rheumatoid arthritis.

Traditional therapies thus see an apparently localised condition like osteoarthritis as an ailment of the whole person and treat it by correcting the surfeit of cold, damp humours.

Gout

Gout is usually included in the "arthritis" group and is an acutely painful disease caused by a build-up of uric acid crystals in the joints (commonly the big toe). It is associated with an inability to break down a group of chemicals called purines that are found in shellfish, red meats and a number of other foods – hence gout's association with over-indulgence and rich food.

Eliminating purine-rich foods from the diet will often reduce symptoms, as will cutting down on fruit sugars (including sweet wines and port). Oxalic acid is another food residue that can build up in the joints, so avoid the rhubarb, sorrel and spinach in which it is found.

Herbal remedies for gout generally contain celery seed, which can help clear excess uric acid from the system. Other useful diuretics and anti-rheumatic plant medicines worth trying include artichoke, carrot, cabbage, cucumber, leek, turnip, stinging nettles, birch, bear's breech and marsh woundwort.

Bruises

A bruise is an area of skin discolouration caused by blood escaping from damaged underlying blood vessels following injury, while a tendency to bruise easily can be related to problems with the blood's ability to clot or may simply suggest that small blood vessels are thin and easily damaged. If your blood does not clot readily – or you are on blood-thinning drugs – avoid taking herbs like feverfew which can slow down clotting still further.

An ice pack in the form of a packet of frozen peas provides an ideal emergency treatment to relieve the pain of a new bruise; better still, keep an ice-cube tray of frozen distilled witch hazel in a plastic bag in the freezer and rub the icy cubes on the affected area instead. Alternating an ice pack with a hot water bottle can help encourage reabsorption of blood and bring more rapid relief. Arnica or comfrey cream applied to unbroken skin will also encourage healing, while if the bruise is the result of some traumatic accident then taking homoeopathic Arnica 6X internally can speed recovery.

Ointments or creams made from daisies or elder leaves were among traditional remedies for bruising and are well worth trying.

Cramp

Cramp is a sudden contraction of the muscles; commonly this occurs in calf muscles which become hard and tense. It can be caused by unusual exercise, stress, tiredness or poor posture, or there may be an imbalance in body salts. In hot weather cramp is often due to a shortage of salt related to dehydration and taking salt tablets can be useful for those prone to cramps. Rubbing the muscle vigorously can bring rapid relief.

Herbal massage oils can be helpful to relax muscles – both marsh woundwort and parsley teas were once popular folk cures for the problem.

Repetitive strain injury

In recent years RSI has become a *cause célèbre* generally associated with using computer keyboards for lengthy periods. In the past similar ailments tended to be categorised by occupation – "upholsterer's hands", "fisherwoman's fingers" and so forth – but any repetitive task, be it typing or playing a musical instrument, can lead to physical problems. RSI often manifests as cramp-like pain or a burning sensation in the hands, arms, shoulders or back, leading ultimately to fatigue, an inability to work effectively and depression.

Baoding balls – Chinese massage balls slightly larger that golf balls – can help. These need to be rotated in the palm for 5-10 minutes each day – a slightly cumbersome skill but one that is not difficult to learn. Start with smaller ping-pong balls if you prefer.

Massage oils containing lavender, thyme, rosemary or eucalyptus can also provide some relief, while internal muscle-relaxing remedies such as nutmeg are worth trying.

Headaches and migraines

Headaches are generally symptoms of some underlying disorder rather than illnesses in their own right. Causes are numerous and the location and character of the pain is often an indication of what that underlying problem might be. Those centred behind the eyes, for example, can suggest a digestive disturbance, while headaches that seem to start at the back of the neck and creep forward are generally tension related. Pain and sensitivity around the eyes or above the nose can be caused by a sinus problem (see page 155).

For some people, tension headaches are extremely common at stressful times; others may find that stress highlights a different area of weakness with stomach upsets or urinary problems. Relaxing herbs such as vervain, skullcap, lavender and St John's wort can ease symptoms, while Siberian ginseng can improve one's stress tolerance and thus reduce the risk of headaches in the first place.

Muscle strain in the shoulders and neck can also contribute to head pain. Sitting or working awkwardly, hunched over a desk or computer keyboard, can easily lead to headaches. Massage oils containing herbs such as thyme, nutmeg, lavender, eucalyptus or juniper rubbed into the affected areas can help prevent headaches developing.

Migraine is an especially common problem and is typically preceded by visual disturbances: jagged lights at the edge of the visual field or a sense that there is a strange out-of-focus area in what one sees. Identifying the cause is again important: this may be food intolerance or stress-related. Red wine, chocolate, pork, citrus fruits, coffee and cheese are all common culprits.

Many sufferers find that chewing feverfew leaves can help prevent attacks, although this herb can cause ulceration of the mucous membranes (usually in the form of mouth ulcers) in sensitive individuals and it should not be taken if this side effect develops. Lavender oil massaged into the temples can sometimes help prevent an attack developing, while valerian and wood betony taken internally can also be useful.

Persistent or sudden unusually severe headaches lasting for three days or more should be referred to a medical practitioner.

Neuralgia

Neuralgia means nerve pain and usually involves an inflammation of the nerve fibres. It can occur anywhere in the body but is most common as an inflammation of the facial or trigeminal nerves which run along the side of the face and scalp. The pain is often exacerbated by cold and draughts and in very severe cases surgical treatment is recommended to cut the nerve.

A useful and often surprisingly effective treatment is simply to dab the area with a little diluted lemon oil or warmed lemon juice; alternatively, try infused St John's wort oil or hot infused chili oil with a few drops of lavender essence added. Internally, nervines such as vervain, oats, skullcap or St John's wort can help, as can circulatory stimulants such as ginger and chili. Jack-by-the-hedge is a traditional remedy for neuralgia and was used in hot poultices.

Assorted inflammations...

Bunions are painful swellings of the joint between the big toe and the adjoining bone which can be caused by badly fitting shoes. Comfortable shoes are essential, while comfrey, marigold or St John's wort creams can ease inflammation and blistering.

Tennis elbow is a painful inflammation of the tendon at the outer edge of the elbow usually caused by excessive exercise — hence the name. As this is an inflammatory problem, herbal anti-inflammatories applied topically can often be helpful. Massage oils containing St John's wort, yarrow or chamomile are worth looking for.

Frozen shoulder is a painful stiffness which can follow injury, stroke or heart attack or may simply develop for no apparent cause. Viewed holistically the problem seems often to be associated with over-controlled anger — the sufferer would unconsciously love to throw a right (or left) hook at someone, but social niceties restrain the motion and the subconscious control leads to stiffness. It can often be helped by remedies which improve liver energy flow — the Chinese associate anger with the liver — so try vervain or self-heal teas as well as external massage rubs containing thyme, yarrow or chamomile oils.

Plants that can help with aches and pains

The following herbs can be helpful — refer to Part 2 for details of use:

Arnica
Birch
Borage
Burdock
Butterbur
Cabbage
Carrot
Celery
Chili
Cloves
Comfrey
Daisy
Devil's claw
Elder
Eucalyptus
Evening primrose
Feverfew
Ginger
Horseradish
Juniper
Lavender
Meadowsweet
Mustard
Olive
Parsley
Pear
Peppermint
Potato
Rosemary
St John's wort
Stinging nettles
Thyme
Turnip
Watercress
Wood betony
Yellow dock

Coughs, colds *and* catarrh

There are still those who at the first hint of a snuffle or sneeze head for their GP's surgery expecting antibiotics to cure the incipient cold overnight. Certainly anti-biotics have a vital role to play in life-threatening diseases, but for common colds and chills herbal remedies can be equally effective. Ancient medical theories often associated illness with climate — and dampness was traditionally associated with phlegm-type diseases such as most coughs and colds.

Common colds and influenza

Today most people believe that colds, flu and coughs are caused by bacteria and viruses. In other ages mysterious "venoms" were to blame, while the Chinese describe colds in terms of attack by external evils — wind, cold, damp, dryness, heat and fire. Whatever the cause there are always some people who will "catch anything going", while others seem to go for years without the slightest hint of a sneeze. Perhaps John Harrison in his book *Love Your Disease* has a point:

The common cold is not a disease, so much as an institution. It is employed skilfully and effectively by those who don't want to be particularly ill but want a period of incapacity. Having achieved that incapacity they can change whatever's troubling them...in this way the common cold or any minor respiratory complaint is used to rebalance the psyche and the internal organs.

In some cases this can well be true and recognising this aspect of a cold is important: curling up in bed with a hot drink or a good book can be a far preferable prescription to antibiotics or patent cold cures.

The typical symptoms of a cold include sore throats, blocked noses, coughs and sneezes. Science blames colds on any one of hundreds of ever-changing viruses: someone who has caught and recovered from a cold can often succumb again, as any immunity to the original virus will be of little use if there is repeated infection.

Because colds are caused by a virus they cannot – despite the optimistic prescriptions – be treated by antibiotics, which are good only for tackling micro-organisms. Orthodox medicine tends to rely on remedies to ease the symptoms, whereas a herbal approach focuses on strengthening the body's immune system and thus helping it to fight the virus. In addition, a number of plants do show anti-viral activity (including lemons and shiitake mushrooms), so can be of real help in countering infection. Frequent colds can be a sign of a weakened immunity – they can also indicate a stressful lifestyle or poor diet and no amount of medicines can solve those.

Combating a cold at the first sign of symptoms is also important. Rather than trying to ignore the increasing catarrh and sore throat until the cold is in full flood, start treatment immediately. Echinacea is one of the best herbs for strengthening the immune system (take three 200 mg capsules or 10 ml of tincture three times daily), while garlic – up to 2 g daily – is especially helpful if the cold develops into a chest infection. Hemp agrimony has also been shown to have good immuno-

stimulant properties and is well worth growing in the garden: summer colds respond well to infusions of fresh hemp agrimony leaves, or the stems can be dried for winter use. Taking up to 5 g of Vitamin C a day can also help. To combat symptoms use anti-catarrhals such as elder flower and yarrow and cut down on refined carbohydrates (sugar and white flour products) as these tend to encourage mucous: eat plenty of fruit – and drink lemon juice – instead.

For feverish chills diaphoretics which encourage sweating are useful: make a decoction of fresh ginger root with a little cinnamon or try elder flower with vervain, meadowsweet and hyssop as an infusion. A popular all-purpose tea for colds is made from equal parts of elder flowers, yarrow and peppermint. This is reasonably palatable and helps to warm the body while having an anti-catarrhal action. In Galenical terms all three herbs are "drying", so would have been used for clearing phlegm in "damp" conditions.

Herbs can also be used in a sympto-matic way for other "cold" problems: for sore throats try gargling with strained and cooled infusions of sage or raspberry leaf, or with lemon juice. A little echinacea tincture added to warm water also makes a good gargle.

Common colds are often labelled as "influenza" but real flu can be severe and in cases life-threatening, with headaches, muscle pain, weakness and high tempera-ture, as well as all the usual symptoms of a bad cold. An attack will typically last for about a week, but will often leave the sufferer feeling depressed and debilitated for some time. Elecampane decoction makes a useful post-influenza tonic – add hyssop if there is a lingering cough or

vervain if depression is severe. Flu can be a particular problem for the elderly, very young, diabetics and those suffering from chronic chest, heart or kidney disorders.

Catarrhal conditions

Modern medicine tends to consider "catarrh" as a uniform problem; however, for the herbalist it can be either "hot" or "cold". Cold catarrh is copious, thin and watery; hot catarrh is thick, scanty and yellow with more inflammation of the mucous membranes. Those with a tendency for "cold" catarrh are often the cold, damp, "phlegmatic" types, with a sluggish digestion. Hot catarrh is a charac-teristic of more active, tense, "choleric" personalities. While cold catarrh is more characteristic of common colds, some types of sinusitis would come into the "hot" category with thick, yellow mucous that stubbornly refuses to move.

Persistent catarrh is extremely common, often seems related to geographic areas (such as damp river valleys) and is associated with a variety of allergies – many of them difficult to avoid, like house dust or car fumes.

Hay fever is associated with pollen allergies in the summer months but the symptoms can be triggered by a range of all-year problems and then become labelled as "allergic rhinitis". Typical symptoms include sneezing, sore and watering eyes, running noses and drowsiness. The physical symptoms are largely due to the body's production of histamine as it attempts to rid itself of the allergen and orthodox treatments are generally based on anti-histamines.

The herbal approach involves strengthening the mucous membranes to help reduce the likely allergic response:

useful herbs include elder flowers, hyssop and golden seal, while anti-allergenic herbs like chamomile and yarrow oils can help reduce symptoms.

Catarrh can stay in the upper respiratory tract, causing nasal congestion, or the mucous can affect the lower airways and be coughed up as phlegm. Lingering catarrh also makes an ideal breeding ground for bacteria and can lead to inflammation of the sinuses – cavities in the bones of the face. Inflammation here can lead to severe pain, made worse by bending forward or blowing the nose.

Sinusitis, with its associated headaches, tooth problems and general discomfort, causes much misery to many people. It is often helped by massaging stimulating ointments containing chili or ginger into the sinus areas above and around the nose. From a holistic point of view sinusitis is often associated with tense personalities who tend to hold their emotions under tight check. Relaxing herbs – such as skullcap or lemon balm – can help, but perhaps the best choice is chamomile. Not only is this a good relaxing nervine, but the combination of heat and water used to make chamomile tea or essential oil, causes anti-inflammatory and anti-spasmodic substances known as azulenes to be produced. Steam inhalations of chamomile flowers are thus good for both the physical effects of sinusitis and its related emotional cause.

While orthodox medicine treats catarrh as a self-contained problem, the condition can also indicate that toxic material elsewhere in the body is not being disposed of adequately   the digestive system could be sluggish or the kidneys not working as efficiently as they should – and cleansing herbs for these areas may solve a persistent catarrhal problem as well.

Whatever the cause, diet is extremely important and, as in the common cold, foods that encourage mucous formation should be avoided. These include refined carbohydrates, dairy products and alcohol. A fruit fast for a couple of days helps to clear any lingering toxic wastes while zinc, garlic and Vitamin C supplements will help to strengthen the immune system and combat infection.

Steam inhalations can also help to clear catarrh. Add 5 drops of thyme or eucalyptus oil to a basin containing a litre of boiling water, cover your head with a towel and inhale the steam for 10 minutes.

Excess catarrh in children can all too frequently lead to ear problems – such as glue ear (see page 162) – and even orthodox researchers now acknowledge that food allergy can be a cause of both middle ear and catarrhal disorders. In trials with 28 patients suffering from *otitis media* (inflammation of the middle ear), 17 people developed nasal symptoms after taking a suspect food, while three-quarters of those also suffered hearing loss or earache as well.

Coughs

Coughing is the body's natural response to any blockage of the airway which may be due to dust and traffic fumes or mucous resulting from infection. Coughing can also be a symptom of a number of more serious illnesses, so professional medical attention is needed for any cough which persists for more than a few days or for which there is no obvious cause.

Coughs can be dry and irritating or "productive" with phlegm which can vary in shade from white to green – darker colours generally indicating an infection. Dry coughs can often linger for weeks following a cold and in some cases coughing can become a nervous habit.

In traditional Chinese medicine the lung is associated with the emotion "grief" and chesty coughs or asthmatic problems can often follow some sort of shock, such as bereavement or redundancy. Remedies for the nervous system, such as lemon balm or St John's wort, can be helpful in these cases.

In all cases, the choice of herbal remedy will depend on the nature of the cough – dry or productive – and whether the phlegm is thick and infected or thin and watery. Herbal cough remedies include expectorants which will encourage the coughing response and the production and excretion of phlegm, and cough suppressants which can ease a persistent dry, tickling cough.

Taking the wrong sort of remedy can do more harm than good. If there is an infection, for example, suppressing the cough and keeping the infected phlegm in the lungs is not a good idea. Equally, if there is no phlegm, taking an expectorant will just make a dry cough more violent. Many herbal expectorants are believed to work by irritating the mucous membranes of the gut, and then, by reflex action (owing to embryonic links between the tissues), also irritating the bronchial membranes so we cough and clear the phlegm. In large doses these herbs are often emetics (that is, they cause vomiting), so taking extra doses in the hope of clearing the cough more rapidly can lead to nausea.

Herbal expectorants are sometimes classified as either "stimulating", which encourage ever more productive coughing, or "relaxing", which have a more soothing effect and loosen phlegm rather than encouraging its violent removal. Elecampane is a stimulating expectorant, while coltsfoot, liquorice, marshmallow and hyssop are relaxing. Raspberry vinegar also helps clear phlegm and adding crushed raspberries to the remedy will improve the flavour.

As well as expectorants and suppressants, herbal cough remedies include demulcents, to soothe irritated mucous membranes, and anti-bacterials to combat infection. Marshmallow, liquorice and plantain are demulcent, while wild lettuce is a cough suppressant.

Suitable antiseptics for chest problems include thyme, which is especially good where the problem is a deep-seated lung infection, and garlic, which can be excreted only through the lungs or skin, so is another good herb for chest infections and one that can be used either as a special "medicine" or simply eaten in lots of very garlicky meals such as *aïoli* or dishes cooked *à la provençale*.

Many cough herbs can be made into syrups – as can onions or leeks – ideally using honey, which is also soothing and healing for the mucous membranes, rather than sugar.

Post-nasal drip – a common cause of coughs – needs an anti-catarrhal approach (see above), but it can also call for expectorants. Hyssop is ideal as it both acts as a gentle, relaxing expectorant and has an anti-catarrhal action. Fennel is also worth considering.

As well as taking cough remedies in teas and syrups, a chest rub can also be useful to help loosen phlegm. The following mixture can be helpful in many cases.

5 drops each of essential oils of fennel and hyssop
10 drops each of essential oils of eucalyptus and thyme

Dilute in 50 ml of carrier oil (e.g. sunflower or almond oil) and massage into the chest two or three times a day. Alternatively, put a few drops of the mixture on a handkerchief and use as an inhalant. A few drops in a saucer of water on the bedside table at night can help relieve night-time congestion.

Sore throats, tonsillitis and laryngitis

Sore throats can be the first sign of a developing cold, although a tendency to "streptococcal throats" – as they are sometimes labelled – can be associated with underlying food allergy and candidiasis. Sore throats can also herald pharyngitis, tonsillitis or German measles with inflammations caused by viral or bacterial infection. As always, if the problem is recurrent, then the cause may be associated with stress (caused by overwork or food intolerance) or a reduced resistance to infection.

This can be especially true with tonsil problems, since these organs are simply small packs of lymphatic tissue at the back of the throat which help protect the body from infection. With children prone to tonsillitis, cutting out milk and milk products and using soya substitutes can often solve otherwise intractable problems. In severe cases the tonsil can become filled with pus, causing an abscess or quinsy which can need urgent surgical treatment, so do not delay in seeking professional help if the problem does not show signs of improvement within 24 hours.

Mild sore throats will often clear in two or three days with or without treatment but the discomfort can be eased by gargles using infusions of herbs like sage, agrimony or raspberry leaf. Alternatively, add 5 ml of tincture to a glass of water – echinacea, thyme or golden seal are effective, although the taste is not pleasant!

Laryngitis is an inflammation of the voice box or larynx and vocal cords usually due to a viral or bacterial infection. It can cause hoarseness or even a complete loss of voice. If symptoms persist for more than a few days then professional investigation is needed in case there is some major problem such as a growth causing the hoarseness. Minor cases can be relieved by gargles (agrimony and echinacea work well, either individually or a mixture of the two) and steam inhalations using thyme, peppermint or eucalyptus oil.

I once had a very severe attack of laryngitis at a herb conference where I had to give what turned out to be an extremely hoarse lecture. Juliette de Baïracli Levy – one of herbalism's *grandes dames* – was also speaking at the event and her recommended cure was certainly my favourite: plenty of ice cream and honey. It didn't instantly restore sound but was very palatable.

Immune weakness

Persistent colds, crops of boils, chronic fatigue or repeated urinary infections, can often indicate reduced resistance. The body's immunity can be stretched by stress, overwork and food allergies, making it harder to combat bacteria, viruses and fungi. Many common organisms are extremely opportunist and while we all harbour numerous potentially lethal bacteria in and on our bodies all the time, if the system is weakened in any way these can very rapidly get out of hand.

Many tonic herbs have a reputation for strengthening the immune system and anyone feeling generally run down or suffering constant minor infections may benefit. Garlic, echinacea and the various types of ginseng have long been used in this way and all are generally best taken for periods of three or four weeks followed by a break. A number of traditional Chinese tonics can also boost the immune system and some are becoming available in the West: the list includes the shiitake mushroom – now available in numerous supermarkets – which is well worth brewing into a soup for those winter days when colds are all too prevalent.

Digestion

There was a saying in medieval Europe to the effect that "death dwells in the bowels" – a belief that good health, or the lack of it, was closely linked to good digestion. In Ayurvedic medicine, digestion plays a similar central role with the *agni*, or digestive fire, responsible for preserving health and numerous remedies used to improve and strengthen this vital energy force.

Modern herbalism, too, puts great emphasis on good digestion with a wide range of herbs to stimulate, relax, normalise and generally improve function. As well as those which have a relaxing and antispasmodic action on the gut, herbal digestive remedies are generally classified as:
• *bitters* – which stimulate the taste receptors leading to increased gastric acid and enzyme production;
• *carminatives* – which help to relieve flatulence, digestive colic and gastric

discomfort by toning the mucous membranes and improving peristalsis;
• *astringents* – which are usually rich in tannins and help to protect mucous membranes while constricting tissues (they will thus help to reduce large bowel overactivity in diarrhoea, for example); and
• *laxatives* – to combat constipation by encouraging bowel motion; these range from the most gentle aperients to violent cathartics which are rarely used these days. Carminatives are often added to combat the griping pains which strong purgatives can cause.

Where digestive remedies are concerned, too, the boundary between food and herbs as medicine grows notably thin. Many culinary herbs are also carminative (such as dill – *Anethum graveolens*, parsley and fennel), warming, bitter stimulants (such as fenugreek – *Trigonella foenum-graecum*) or antispasmodics like the mints and rosemary; the French, who seem to have a national preoccupation with the

Plants that can help with colds, coughs and catarrh		
The following herbs can be helpful – refer to Part 2 for details of use:		
	Daisy	Liquorice
	Echinacea	Marshmallow
	Elder	Meadowsweet
	Elecampane	Mustard
	Eucalyptus	Onion
Apricot	Fig	Peppermint
Beetroot	Garlic	Plantain
Bitter orange	Ginger	Raspberry
Borage	Golden seal	Shiitake mushrooms
Burdock	Horseradish	Slippery elm
Butterbur	Hyssop	Thyme
Chili	Jack-by-the-hedge	Turnip
Cinnamon	Leek	Valerian
Coltsfoot	Lemon	Yarrow
Common mallow	Lettuce	Yellow dock
Creeping Jenny	Linden	

state of their livers, will regularly eat dandelion leaves, which have liver-toning properties, as salad.

According to the Chinese, the liver governs the smooth flow of vital energy or *Qi* through the body, it also stores blood, governs the tendons and is linked with the eyes and poor vision: itching or dry eyes are often associated with liver disharmonies. The Chinese say that the liver "stores the soul" – governing spirit and mental activity: weak liver energy can thus lead to emotional disorders, depression or mental sluggishness. A wide range of apparently disparate symptoms can therefore be linked to basic liver imbalances, so eating herbs (or foods) which help to stimulate the liver – such as artichoke, asparagus and cabbage – can often improve general health as well.

Constipation

If concern over their livers is a national preoccupation for the French, then the bowels fulfil the same role for the British: we spend millions of pounds each year on over-the-counter laxatives in an effort to keep "regular". Many of these laxatives work by irritating the bowel to encourage peristalsis: long-term misuse damages the bowel mucosa and weakens the gut, leading to problems like diverticulosis.

There is no "standard pattern" or "normal" bowel movements. Some people go every day, others every other day or twice a day. Diet is, obviously, significant, with vegetarians and those eating a high-fibre diet likely to have a more frequent pattern of bowel motions than those eating mainly meat and refined carbohydrates. The food we eat also influences how long it can take to be excreted: for traditional people in the Third World it

may take about 12 hours or less for food to pass through, whereas for those eating a conventional Western diet it can be as long as 72 hours.

Low-fibre diet combined with a lack of exercise – and often coupled with a sluggish lifestyle or personality – leads to what is sometimes called "flaccid" or "atonic" constipation. Constipation can also be associated with nervous tension and a hectic lifestyle with little time to respond to the normal urge to defecate. The sufferer is often so stressed that the digestive system is unable to relax and allow normal function to progress. In such cases stools are sometimes described as resembling rabbit droppings. This type of constipation can alternate with bouts of diarrhoea and may lead to the catch-all label of "irritable bowel syndrome" (see below).

Atonic constipation can be helped by exercise, a high-fibre diet (or the use of a bulking laxative such as isphaghula) and abdominal massage. Stronger herbal laxatives – such as the well known senna pods (*Senna alexandrina*) – contain chemicals called anthraquinones and work by irritating the bowel. Bilberries, carrots, figs, grapes, liquorice, olives, pears and walnuts are all rather gentler in action, but can still be helpful at combating constipation.

For constipation associated with nervous tension, bowel relaxants such as chamomile and lemon balm can be worth adding to the mixture. Gentle sources of fibre are preferable in this type of constipation, so conventional "roughage" – such as bran – should often be avoided, as should the anthraquinone herbs. Relaxation and a general reduction in stress levels are also important.

Irritable bowel syndrome

Stress and anxiety can also play a part in another common disorder, "irritable bowel syndrome" – a name that is often little more than a convenient label for a range of symptoms that can embrace just about any bowel irregularity which does not have a clear pathological cause. Sufferers can complain of numerous problems typical of poor digestive function or food intolerance – including constipation, diarrhoea, bloating, flatulence, stomach cramps, nausea, bowel tenderness, headaches, general tiredness, depression or anxiety. Food intolerance is a common cause: one study suggests that two-thirds of IBS sufferers actually display some sort of food allergy. The main culprits include dairy food, gluten (found in wheat, oats, barley and rye), caffeine-containing drinks, alcohol, cigarettes, eggs and red meat. If food intolerance is the cause, then it is important to identify and avoid the problem categories.

Soothing herbs such as marshmallow and meadowsweet can help to relieve IBS symptoms, as can digestive tonics and stimulants like peppermint and golden seal. Astringents, such as herb Robert and agrimony, can be added to these remedies to ease any symptoms of diarrhoea.

Many women find that irritable bowel symptoms get worse just before a period and a clinical trial at Addenbroke's Hospital in Cambridge used evening primrose oil on sufferers. The researchers based their project on the fact that excess production of certain sorts of prostaglandins (PGE_2) has been linked to certain types of IBS. *Gamma-linolenic acid* – found in evening primrose and borage oils – can influence which sorts of prostaglandins are produced and the study demonstrated that large doses of the oil (3-4 g daily) for at least three months brought significant improvements in IBS when it was related to pre-menstrual problems.

Diarrhoea

Nervous tension is a common cause of an over-active digestive tract and problems with diarrhoea – although there are plenty of other causes too: infection from bacteria, chills, over-eating, alcohol or other irritant foods can all cause problems. Excessive bowel motions can lead to cramping pains and general soreness in the anal area, while the associated symptoms can include nausea and vomiting.

Sudden diarrhoea is most commonly caused by some sort of gastro-intestinal infection – especially if others who shared the same meal are similarly affected. This is an all-too-common problem for holidaymakers who may find that local standards of hygiene in exotic locations are not quite the same as back home. When travelling in high-risk areas never eat raw salads, always wash and peel fruit, avoid ice cubes in drinks and regard street-side hawkers selling "bottled water" with some suspicion.

In Chinese medicine, fruits and salads are regarded as "cooling" or *yin* in character and an excess can thus lead to stomach chills and diarrhoea problems – much as Gerard warned against eating cucumbers in winter. Leaving our cold northern isle (*yin* in character) and heading for sunny holiday spots to eat all those exotic fruits can upset the *yin-yang* balance and can contribute just as much

to holiday tummy upsets as poor hygiene.

Diarrhoea and vomiting are the body's natural reaction to an infecting organism and are often the best way of getting rid of it quickly: herbal treatment helps with astringent remedies to soothe the digestive tract. Strong, cold, black Indian tea – without milk or sugar – is rich in tannins and can ease an over-worked gut if nothing better is available.

Gastric flu and stomach chills can also lead to diarrhoea. Again symptoms are likely to be short-lived and using astringent herbal mixtures (such as agrimony, herb Robert or marigold) combined with anti-infection herbs like echinacea or hemp agrimony can help. Diarrhoea is very dehydrating and it is important to increase fluid intake during such bouts – especially with babies and small children

Regular diarrhoea is more likely to be stress-related. This can range from the irritating, but largely harmless, increased frequency before exams or job interviews, to debilitating disorders such as ulcerative colitis which require professional attention and can lead to long-term, chronic illness. Sedating herbs – such as chamomile, lemon balm or skullcap – can help.

Piles

Constipation is often associated with piles, or haemorrhoids – a type of varicose veins which can easily be felt, like bunches of grapes, around the rectum. Minor cases can often be cured completely, although once formed piles do have a tendency to recur later in life and can often be rekindled by over-exertion as well as by recurrent bouts of constipation. Pilewort is an obvious

remedy, although ointments of many astringent herbs – including witch hazel, marigold and agrimony – can also help.

Stomach upsets and gastritis

Minor stomach upsets with abdominal pain, nausea, diarrhoea and vomiting affect most of us at some time. They can often be associated with food poisoning (see above), an excess of rich food or too much alcohol; in such cases soothing herbs like slippery elm and marshmallow can bring relief. Other stomach upsets are linked to chills, when warming herbs such as chili and ginger can be useful.

For some, the problem can be stress related, with any increase in nervous tension or anxiety levels usually accompanied by digestive problems; relaxing carminatives can be useful in these cases. The wide range of herbal relaxants offers plenty of choice depending on individual need and tastes, but a good mixture for nervous tummies is:

2 parts chamomile flowers
2 parts lemon balm herb
1 part lavender flowers

Use 1-2 teaspoons of dried mixed herbs per cup of boiling water, infuse for 5 minutes, strain and drink.

Nervousness can be one cause of gastric over-activity with excess acid production leading to gastritis or inflammation of the stomach lining. Eventually such damage can lead to ulceration. Other causes of gastritis include over-indulgence in rich foods and alcohol with symptoms similar to those of food poisoning – nausea, vomiting and diarrhoea. Those prone to gastritis should avoid irritant foods – spices, tea, coffee, alcohol, fried foods and pickles – and eat smaller meals more regularly.

An orthodox approach will generally concentrate on antacids to reduce stomach acid, but this can simply encourage even more acid production in an attempt to normalise the digestive process. Herbal remedies will generally include soothing mucilages and anti-inflammatories with herbs that will cover and protect the stomach lining and encourage healing. Slippery elm is popular in over-the-counter remedies and is available in tablets or as powder which simply needs mixing with water. Other possibilities include meadowsweet, liquorice, chamomile and marshmallow.

Indigestion

There are numerous possible causes of indigestion, including rushed meals, wearing tight belts, eating irregularly or while feeling tense, and too many rich or potentially irritant foods. The result is a mixture of heartburn, pain in the lower chest, flatulence and nausea that goes under the label of dyspepsia.

Herbal solutions include relaxing plants such as chamomile and lemon balm to help to reduce the anxiety and tension which can contribute to indigestion, and aromatic carminatives such as fennel, peppermint or ginger to ease flatulence and nausea. Meadow-sweet and slippery elm, can help to protect the stomach from high acid secretions, while bitter remedies such as artichoke, bitter orange or cornflower will help to stimulate the digestive process and restore normal function without focusing on stomach acidity.

Heartburn can be a particular problem in chronic obesity and pregnancy where the stomach is forced upwards and the muscle which divides the oesophagus from the stomach is weakened and may eventually lead to a hiatus hernia. Symptoms are often worse at night as there is nothing to stop acid leaking into the oesophagus when sufferers are lying down. Raising the head of the bed by 10–15 cm by putting normal house bricks under the legs will prevent acid leaking out of the stomach and can prove a very simple way of reducing symptoms. Slippery elm and marshmallow, either combined in capsules or mixed as powders with a little water to form a paste, make a useful combination for regular heartburn and are also safe to take in pregnancy.

The pain of indigestion can be confused with heart pain from disorders like angina pectoris. This sort of pain eases with rest, while heartburn is generally worse when the sufferer lies down. Sudden severe "indigestion" in someone who has previously been symptom free should always be investigated professionally for a possible underlying heart condition. Chronic indigestion can also be a sign of peptic ulcers, gall bladder disorders, liver problems or cancer; expert diagnosis is essential.

An aspect of indigestion is wind – up or down – which is usually more of an embarrassment than an indicator of serious health problems. As the Galenical practitioners knew only too well, certain foods are windy – beans and the brassica family are common culprits. To combat wind from such cold, damp foods, the medieval housewife added warming

spices like pepper and ginger. Including fennel, dill, rosemary or sage in our cooking not only improves the flavour but also adds herbs to stimulate and soothe the digestive system and reduce that risk of wind and indigestion.

Nausea and vomiting

Nausea and vomiting can be associated with a wide range of illnesses: from life-threatening fevers and stomach problems to motion sickness, pregnancy, migraines and indigestion. It is important to seek professional help for severe and persistent problems, but minor disorders, with a clear cause, can easily be helped by herbal remedies at home.

For nausea associated with stomach upsets herbs such as lemon balm, bitter orange, dandelion or marshmallow can be helpful.

Travel sickness – whether it occurs in trains, planes, shops or cars – is especially prevalent among children and soon becomes a problem for the entire family. Symptoms start with pallor, sweating and nausea and lead to vomiting and, sometimes, fainting. The disorder is generally to do with the delicate balance mechanism in the inner ear, and since children's ears tend to be more sensitive the problem is more commonplace among the young.

The best herbal remedy for all types of nausea is ginger – in capsules, tinctures or even in the form of sweets, ginger drinks and biscuits. Ginger beer is ideal for children; alternatively, travel with a small dropper bottle of ginger tincture and simply put a few drops on the tongue before the journey and as needed during the trip.

Plants that can help with digestive problems

The following herbs can be helpful – refer to Part 2 for details of use:

Agrimony
Apple
Artichoke
Asparagus
Bear's breech
Beetroot
Bilberry
Bitter orange
Borage
Buchu
Burdock
Butterbur
Cabbage
Carrot
Chamomile
Chili
Cinnamon
Cloves
Coffee
Coltsfoot
Comfrey
Common mallow
Cornflower

Creeping Jenny
Cucumber
Daisy
Dandelion
Devil's claw
Echinacea
Elecampane
Evening primrose
Fennel
Feverfew
Garlic
Ginger
Ginseng
Golden seal
Grape
Greater celandine
Hawthorn
Herb Robert
Hops
Horseradish
Hyssop
Isphaghula
Lavender
Lettuce
Linden
Liquorice
Marigold
Marshmallow

Meadowsweet
Mustard
Nutmeg
Onion
Parsley
Pear
Peppermint
Pineapple
Potato
Purple loosestrife
Raspberry
Sage
Self-heal
Shepherd's purse
Shiitake mushrooms
Skullcap
Strawberries
Tea
Thyme
Toadflax
Tomato
Vervain
White deadnettle
Witch hazel
Wood avens
Wood betony
Yellow dock

Eyes *and* ears

Herbs have a long history of use in treating eye and ear problems: before the days of universally available hearing aids and spectacles, itinerant herb doctors would often specialise in eyes or ears and travel the countryside treating patients with brews designed to improve sight or hearing rather than simply alleviate the sort of minor ailments we would treat in this way today.

Old herbals are full of remedies – the vast majority unproven – for restoring sight to the blind and curing tinnitus or deafness. Some, such as the legend about greater celandine seeds restoring sight to blind swallows, go back to ancient times and were once very widely used. Other remedies we now know do have a relevance: eating carrots certainly has a role in improving night vision, since Vitamin A is needed to maintain the relevant components in the retina.

In Chinese theory the eyes are associated with the liver and the ears with the kidneys. They are links which one can well understand: excess alcohol, for example, usually leads to an overworked liver and sluggish, bleary eyes. Traditionally, too, the kidney is the home of the body's "reproductive energy" which inevitably runs down as we reach middle age and the menopause. As we get older hearing problems become more commonplace so, again, it is understandable how these connections were first formulated.

This traditional approach can be effective: in China, for example, chrysanthemums (see page 111) are used to treat various liver complaints and are also recommended for eye weaknesses, while herbs which warm the kidneys – such as buchu and cinnamon – can be usefully added to remedies for earache and other weaknesses.

For home use, however, it is best to limit the use of herbal remedies to minor, self-limiting conditions: eyes and ears are sensitive and precious and using impure or crude remedies can do more harm than good.

Eye problems

Blepharitis is an inflammation of the eyelid which can be caused by an allergic reaction to cosmetics and is often accompanied by white scales on the lashes. In chronic cases the eyelid can become ulcerated with a yellow crust, the eyelashes are often matted and may fall out. Use eye-baths made by decocting marigold petals and then thoroughly straining the mixture (to ensure that it is sterile and clean). Allow the decoction to cool thoroughly and then bathe the eye every few hours.

Conjunctivitis, also known as red eye, is an inflammation of the fine membrane (conjunctiva) covering the eyeball. Sufferers usually complain of severe pain, watering and a "gritty feeling" on blinking. Again, a well-strained decoction of marigold is normally recommended for use as an eye-bath, but decoctions of herb Robert or toadflax can be used in similar ways.

Styes are an acute inflammation of a gland at the base of an eyelash usually caused by bacterial infection. They can indicate lowered resistance due to stress, overwork or repeated infection. A little marigold cream or tea tree cream can be applied to the site of infection, but take great care not to smudge the creams into the eye itself as they can sting. Alternatively, use the same sorts of astringent and antiseptic decoctions suggested for conjunctivitis. Taking garlic or echinacea internally can help combat the infection and improve immunity.

Tired eyes: We've all suffered from sore, tired eyes after too much reading or too much time spent in a highly polluted atmosphere: close the eyes and cover with slices of cucumber or used tea-bags of green tea or chamomile.

Ear problems

Earache is common, extremely painful and distressing (especially in children) and needs great care in treating as infection can lead to perforated eardrums and the risk of permanent hearing damage. The cause is usually an acute local infection, which can be related to sinus or catarrhal problems, and use of anti-catarrhals and suitable steam inhalants (see page 155) can help. If there is any discharge or possibility that the ear drum has burst then seek immediate medical help. For minor cases ear drops using infused oils of mullein (*Verbascum thapsus*) or St John's wort flowers are safe for home use. Put a few drops in the ear and then insert a cotton-wool plug. Repeat three or four times a day as needed. Massaging the mastoid bone (behind the ear) with antiseptic oils such as lavender and tea

tree can also help. A traditional cure was to insert the heart of a freshly boiled onion into the ear – a suitably hot and ideally shaped healing poultice if nothing else is available.

Glue ear is common in children and involves an inflammation of the middle ear (*otitis media*) with a build-up of fluid leading to deafness. It is often associated with food allergy and can improve significantly if the sufferer tries a milk-free diet. Orthodox treatment usually involves surgery to insert grommets into the eardrum to relieve the fluid pressure; these generally have to be replaced after a few months as they tend to fall out. Anti-catarrhals such as golden seal and ribwort plantain taken internally can often help.

Tinnitus – an irritating whistling and rattling sound affecting one or both ears – can be caused by nerve damage (common in those who work in noisy environments) or labyrinth disorders like Ménières disease. Some argue it is associated with stress, anger and psychological problems and will disappear once sufferers learn to relax and solve their emotional disturbances. This can sometimes be true, especially where there is no apparent pathological cause, but in cases involving nerve damage is generally not so. Some suggest that the noise is related to the sound of blood flow around the ears and ginkgo has been variously reported to help the problem by improving cerebral circulation. Wood betony has similar properties. These remedies can be worth trying, as can Chinese kidney tonics such as cinnamon or even the traditional cures of drinking plenty of beetroot juice and eating leeks: occasionally the result is significant improvement – but tinnitus is a stubborn condition and there is often no easy solution.

Plants that can help with eyes and ears

The following herbs can be helpful – refer to Part 2 for details of use:

Beetroot
Carrot
Cornflower
Cucumber
Dandelion
Ginkgo
Herb Robert
Leek
Onion
Shepherd's purse
Toadflax
Walnut
Witch hazel

Heart and circulation

Today, thanks to modern science, we generally regard the heart simply as a powerful muscle to pump blood around the body. Traditional medicine has a rather different view: to the Chinese the heart controls the life process, co-ordinates the activities of all the other organs and manages mental activities and consciousness. It stores *Shen* – a sense of appropriateness and right behaviour – so that what we term mental illness is often seen in Chinese medicine as due to disharmonies in the heart upsetting *Shen*.

Ayurvedic medicine puts the heart in a similar central role: it is the dwelling place of the *atman* – the divine self or spirit of immortal life – controlling consciousness and affected by spiritual weakness. Western Ayurvedic experts like David Frawley argue that the high level of heart disease in Western society is due to our over-preoccupation with personal achievement and material wealth – we die of "spiritual starvation", causing a broken heart.

Like modern allopathic medicine, much Western herbalism is rather more concerned with symptomatic relief of cardiovascular problems than with the spiritual aspects of the heart and few would consider heart problems as suitable candidates for home remedies. Self-help is, however, possible – either from an orthodox standpoint using herbs to improve circulation or reduce cholesterol levels or adopting a more traditional approach and feeding the heart on more spiritual remedies.

High blood pressure

Until the invention of the sphygno-manometer we had no accurate way of measuring blood pressure and so problems with high blood pressure passed under a variety of other names. Today, DIY blood-pressure machines seem to have taken over from the "speak your weight" scales that used to lurk on every railway station and passers-by can be suitably terrified by instant readings which declare them to be "high". Isolated blood pressure readings really mean very little: several consistently high ones are needed before applying the label "hypertension" and mild cases can often be controlled by simple dietary measures.

Coffee, for example, contains caffeine which stimulates the heart to beat faster, pumping blood through the vessels and kidneys more energetically. The result – even in the healthy – can be an abnormally fast pulse, irregular heart beat, raised blood pressure and increased desire to urinate. Often simply cutting down on coffee – along with tea and chocolate, which contain similar chemicals – is all that is needed.

Herbal infusions make an ideal alternative for those prone to hypertension: use relaxing or mildly hypotensive herbs such as skullcap, passion flower, celery seed, yarrow, vervain, hawthorn, self-heal, valerian or linden flowers. Diuretics can also help if the heart's performance is weak and fluids tend to accumulate in the system. Dandelion leaf is ideal because it contains a good supply of potassium which can be lost when urination is increased by the use of diuretics. A typical infusion for raised blood pressure is:

2 parts hawthorn flowers
2 parts lime flowers
1 part dandelion leaf
1 part yarrow
1 part vervain

One teaspoon of the mixture infused with a cup of boiling water to be taken two or three times a day.

Modern advice for maintaining a healthy heart usually includes cutting down on fatty foods which could increase the blood's cholesterol levels. Cholesterol is a complex fatty substance which is essential for physical health. The average body contains about 150 g of the stuff and it plays an important role in maintaining membrane fluidity, as well as providing the raw material for manufacturing many hormones and bile acids. This useful substance can, unfortunately, encourage fatty deposits to develop in blood vessels, which in turn leads to hardening of the arteries and increased blood pressure. Numerous herbs can help to reduce the levels of cholesterol in the blood and encourage its excretion; much research has focused on garlic, which has been proven to help reduce the risk of a further heart attack in those already suffering problems with cardiovascular damage and atherosclerosis. Daily doses of 1-4 cloves per person have been suggested as ideal – which is no more than one could easily use in cooking. German trials suggest that 2 g a day of powdered garlic is sufficient to achieve notable therapeutic effects.

Other foodstuffs which have been shown to have a similar cholesterol-lowering action include chickpeas, kidney beans, navy beans (the sort that go into cans of baked beans), lentils, soya beans and alfalfa sprouts. Useful cholesterol-lowering herbs include nutmeg, sage, linden, thyme, garlic, liquorice and ginseng. Also important is tea: research suggests that green and oolong teas are the most effective at lowering cholesterol levels. Traditionally the oolong tea *Pu Erh* has been regarded as a good digestive remedy after rich meals. In the early 1980s French researchers reported a reduction of 25% in cholesterol blood levels in a group of high risk patients after a month of *Pu Erh* drinking. The tea needs to be taken without milk, since milk precipitates the tannins which are believed to be mainly responsible for this cholesterol-lowering property.

Circulatory problems and chilblains

Poor heart function can contribute to numerous circulation problems which may include severe pain in the legs while walking (intermittent claudication) and Buerger's disease (common among heavy smokers); this can eventually lead to gangrene and necessitate amputation.

Among more minor circulation problems are chilblains, which are generally associated not with failing hearts but with cold, as the body responds to falling temperatures by constricting blood supply to the peripheries in order to keep vital organs and deep tissues warm.

Wearing adequate clothing on cold days is the easiest way to avoid occasional chilblains, while habitual sufferers can improve their circulation with stimulating herbs like ginger, cinnamon, horseradish and chili. Recent research suggests that ginkgo can improve the peripheral blood circulation, although it is more traditionally regarded as stimulating the blood supply to the brain.

Arnica cream can help relieve the discomfort of chilblains once they've appeared, but should not be used on broken skin. Other helpful herbs to relieve symptoms include aloe vera and pot marigold. Warming herbs such as ginger, cinnamon or chili can be helpful if circulation is generally weak – especially in the elderly.

Anaemia

While science has simplified the heart's role to that of pump, we now know that blood chemistry is extremely complex and the cause of numerous disorders. Iron-deficient anaemia is one of the most common and is widespread among women of child-bearing age.

The traditional Western herbal approach includes adding numerous iron-rich foods to the diet – such as apricots, asparagus, beetroot, carrots, stinging nettle and watercress – while the Chinese concentrate on herbs which help ''nourish'' or manufacture blood. One of the most popular is *Dang Gui* (*Angelica polymorpha* var. *sinensis*), which is now widely available in prepackaged, over-the-counter products from health food shops and chemists. It is useful for anaemia as well as various menstrual disorders, and contains Vitamin B_{12} and folic acid, which can counter some types of anaemia.

Varicose veins

Varicose veins are usually visible as tortuous, knotted veins on the surface of the legs. They can ache or the surrounding area can be prone to swelling. The flesh surrounding the affected area can often feel hot.

Veins, unlike arteries, have to help force blood back to the heart rather than depend on the impetus of this powerful pump. The muscles surrounding deep veins can help considerably, but the superficial veins in the legs often have little support for forcing blood back to the central pumping system and over the years they can become distended, lengthened and tortuous.

Deep breathing can help encourage the return of blood from the peripheries while a tendency to varicose veins can often be countered by each morning alternately hosing the legs with a hot and cold shower, several times, for 1-2 minutes each time. Using bricks to raise the end of the bed to aid venous return at night can also help. Useful external treatments include distilled witch hazel, lemon juice, infusions of vine leaf, agrimony or pilewort and fig poultices.

Varicose ulcers generally occur in the elderly and are associated with poor circulation, with reduced blood flow to an area often making healing difficult. Professional treatment is usually essential, but using infused oils containing heating herbs like chili and ginger as a gentle massage around the ulcer (not on it) can help stimulate blood flow to the area to encourage healing.

Internally herbs which contains flavonoids and coumarins – chemicals known to strengthen blood vessels and also reduce the risk of clots – may be helpful. Traditional specific remedies include horsechestnut (*Aesculus hippo-castanum*) and melilot (*Melilotus officinalis*, also known as king's clover). Herbs like rue (*Ruta graveolens*) and buckwheat (*Fagopyrum esculentum*) are high in rutin (a flavonoid) which can help to strengthen blood vessels.

Plants that can help with heart and circulation	
The following herbs can be helpful – refer to Part 2 for details of use:	
	Hawthorn
	Lemon
	Linden
	Marigold
	Oats
Apple	Olive
Arnica	Onion
Borage	Passion flower
Celery	Self-heal
Fig	Shepherd's purse
Garlic	Siberian ginseng
Ginkgo	Skullcap
Ginseng	Valerian
Golden seal	Walnut
Grape	Yarrow

Mouth disorders

In Chinese theory the mouth is associated with the spleen – an organ traditionally linked with digestion, so red, lustrous lips suggest that food is being well digested and assimilated, while pale lips indicate poor spleen energy with a weak appetite and abnormal digestion. The condition of the gums, too, is indicative of the state of the digestion: red, swelling and bleeding gums indicate excess stomach heat, as do mouth ulcers around the lips. Mouth problems are thus often related to other bodily ills and should rarely be considered in isolation.

Bad breath

Bad breath, too, can suggest digestive upsets: it can accompany constipation or gastritis or may simply be the result of eating highly spiced foods or garlic, smoking or tooth decay.

One of the traditional remedies to sweeten the breath is chewing fennel seeds – they have a pleasant aniseed flavour and the same seeds were once also recommended to stave off hunger pains during lengthy Sunday morning sermons. Sucking peppermints is a common choice for bad breath, but peppermint sweets are generally high in sugar, which is damaging for the teeth, while too much peppermint oil can be irritant on the mucous membranes of mouth, upper respiratory tract and stomach.

Using an unsweetened herbal infusion as a mouthwash is a good way of combating mouth infections and tooth decay: try sage, thyme or rosemary. Chewing parsley leaves can often help to reduce garlic smells.

If the problem is associated with stagnation in the digestive tract, with food taking too long to pass through, then gentle laxative remedies, like yellow dock, or liver stimulants, like toadflax or dandelion, can be useful as well.

Gum disease

Gum disease is, fortunately, not as commonplace as it once was thanks to better oral hygiene and a more positive approach to conservative dentistry.

Brushing regularly and correctly is important, as is eating foods which contain roughage and can help clean the teeth as they are chewed. The traditional "apple a day" is an extremely effective herbal remedy, as is a piece of cheese (without biscuits) after a meal or – even better – a cup of unsweetened green tea at the end of a meal: this is rich in fluoride and has been shown to prevent tooth decay.

Herbal mouthwashes can help with minor problems of localised bleeding or inflamed gums – infusions of sage, agrimony or marigold can all be effective.

Mouth ulcers

Mouth ulcers – or aphtha – commonly start with a sore red patch of blisters erupting to produce a greyish white ulcer. They will usually clear of their own accord after a week or so, but can be so painful that eating becomes almost impossible.

No one really knows why mouth ulcers occur: the Chinese blame stomach heat but others maintain they are due to low-grade fungal infections, excess sugar or may indicate a weakened immune system. Recurrent bouts of mouth ulcers can suggest some underlying weakness

and a course of immune-stimulant herbs and tonics can help: taking garlic or ginseng for a month can boost the system. Herbal mouthwashes using sage, birch, cloves, rosemary or echinacea can help relieve symptoms.

Plants that can help with mouth problems

The following herbs can be helpful – refer to Part 2 for details of use:

Birch
Cloves
Daisy
Fennel
Feverfew
Grape
Greater celandine
Linden
Rosemary
Sage
Self-heal
Wood avens

Nervous disorders, anxiety and stress

While a certain amount of stress is essential to keep us alert and active, an excess is probably one of the most pervasive ills of the late 20th century. We live in an age in which people frequently describe themselves as "time poor, cash rich" – in other words, too busy working and earning to spend much time relaxing and enjoying life.

Taking soothing remedies is only a small part of the solution. Many of the ills caused by stress could be solved with a little relaxation – time spent on learning to relax with yoga or Tai Ch'i classes or going for unhurried rambles in the fresh air. Instead of resting on the seventh day we spend it in supermarket queues, endless home improvements or catching up with the housework. We all – even the busiest parent – need to find space for ourselves each day in order to cope and a few minutes of relaxed deep breathing or listening to a favourite piece of music will work wonders.

An holistic approach always focuses on the needs of body, mind and spirit and this is especially true with any condition labelled as "nerves". Physical manifestations of "nervous disorders" may include insomnia, palpitations or headaches; emotional aspects can include irritability, depression, feelings of anger or guilt while the lack of determination, emptiness or sense of purpose felt by so many people can typify the spiritual vacuum at the centre of many modern lifestyles.

Herbs can be equally holistic, operating on the same three levels to improve well-being: vervain is a good example. It can be considered as a liver tonic and relaxing nervine. Taken in Bach Flower Remedy form (see page 169) it is suitable for the perfectionist, slightly obsessional personality who tries to do too many jobs at once and runs each task to death, like a dog worrying a bone. On a spiritual level vervain can increase understanding and psychic awareness: it was once used in scrying and some maintain that it will repair holes in the human aura (a layer of psychic energy which surrounds all living things and is seen in Kirlian photography).

In Chinese and Ayurvedic medicine emotional imbalance is well accepted as a possible cause of physical disease: the Chinese associate the emotion "fear" with the kidneys, for example, and panic attacks could be a sign of kidney imbalance. "Anger" can have a similar effect on the liver, while what the Chinese describe as "joy" (but may be better translated as "over-enthusiasm") can lead to heart disorders.

Herbal nervines work on several levels, including:

• herbal sedatives and relaxants which can ease tensions, feelings of anxiety or help with insomnia;
• herbal tonics and stimulants which will provide an additional short-term energy boost; and
• herbal remedies which can act on the emotions or spirit in some way as part of a total holistic approach.

They can be used much as orthodox sedatives, hypnotics or anti-depressants: skullcap is a sedative, for example, passion flower a hypnotic – to dull the senses or induce sleep – and St John's wort a

potent anti-depressant. Such herbal remedies should not, however, be seen as a complete alternative to professional counselling or psychotherapy for those who really cannot cope with their lifestyles.

Anxiety and tension

Taking the time to brew a relaxing herbal tea and then do nothing but sit, sip it and unwind is a far more therapeutic way of combating tension than popping a couple of tranquillisers and carrying on with the normal frenetic daily routine. Suitable herbs to add into the relaxing brew include lemon balm, skullcap, chamomile, wood betony, valerian and vervain.

Herbal baths are equally effective: use either 500 ml of an infusion of a highly aromatic relaxing herb – such as chamomile, lavender or lemon balm – or else a few drops of the essential oil.

Tension often leads to headaches as the muscles at the back of the neck stiffen. Massaging that area and the temples can help: use lavender oil diluted in a vegetable-oil base. A 50:50 combination of wood betony and lavender as an infusion is another good remedy for tension headaches, although it is always best to take the tea as soon as symptoms start to appear rather than waiting for a major headache to develop.

Anxiety and worries can lead to depression and unhappiness. Severe depression needs professional help but for minor "downs" lemon balm and borage can be especially uplifting, while St John's wort is gaining in reputation as equivalent in effect to many orthodox drugs. These herbs can also be supportive for those undergoing professional treatment.

Old herbals often describe how even looking on cheerful plants can lift the spirits and "comfort the harte". Perhaps it is worth remembering part of an old Persian poem:

If of thy mortal goods thou art bereft,
And of thy store, three loaves alone
*   are left,*
Sell one, and with the dole
Buy hyacinths to feed the soul.

Insomnia

The amount of sleep we each need varies considerably and sometimes we require rather more sleep than at others. Sleeplessness only becomes a problem when sufferers feel tired and unable to concentrate during the day or when it becomes a worry in itself. There are many causes for disturbed sleep patterns: heavy meals late at night can lead to disturbed digestion; painful joints and muscles or irritating coughs will keep most people awake, while catnapping during the day simply fills up the sleep quota and there is no need for further rest.

Insomnia is commonly associated with tension, worries and a failure to relax before bedtime. The majority of herbal remedies for sleeplessness are based on sedative and relaxing herbs which will help to reduce anxieties, calm an over-active mind and encourage sleep. Unlike orthodox treatments they are non-addictive, although some people find that the potency of an insomnia remedy is reduced if they take it regularly, so it can be worthwhile changing the mix from time to time if long-term use is likely.

As always with herbal medicine, it is far better to identify and treat the cause of a problem rather than simply tackle the symptoms, so if inability to relax or over-anxiety is the root cause of insomnia, meditation classes or a review of lifestyle concerns might provide the solution. Vervain taken in its Bach Flower Remedy form (see page 169) can be particularly useful for such tense individuals. Other suitable remedies include hops, wild lettuce, passion flower or Californian poppy.

Improving energy levels

Herbal stimulants are, of course, familiar to all: coffee, tea and chocolate which are rich in caffeine, theobromine and related alkaloids and are regularly used as a short-term restorative to keep students and night owls awake. They are, however, superficial remedies offering no real long-term benefits when it comes to improving energy levels and strengthening the nervous system. A better alternative is rosemary, which contains a stimulant called borneal. Take it as an infusion or add a few drops of rosemary oil to stimulating baths.

Longer-term energy tonics are often a better option: Korean ginseng is now well established in the West as a tonic remedy. In traditional Chinese medicine, ginseng tends to be regarded as boosting the masculine (*yang*) energies and, while it can be taken by women, other tonics are often preferable. Siberian ginseng is traditionally feminine (*yin*) in character and so can be more suitable for women. A favourite Chinese tonic for women is *Dang Gui* (see page 164), now more widely available in the West. Other tonic herbs worth considering include shiitake mushrooms, elecampane, oats, almonds, grapes, thyme, liquorice and sage.

If a stressful time is looming – such as exams or a heavy work period – then it is worth taking tonic herbs before the event to provide an energy boost, rather than depending on short-term stimulants once the stresses mount. Siberian ginseng is particularly useful for helping the body cope more efficiently with stress and improving performance: it was widely used in the 1960s and '70s by Soviet athletes and long-distance lorry-drivers to increase stamina.

Mind and spirit

Western practitioners often avoid discussions of spirituality which, like death, is one of our 20th-century taboo subjects. Using herbs such as shiitake mushrooms can help to strengthen the spirit and give a patient the will and self-determination to make the major lifestyle changes essential for long-term recovery. A few drops of rose oil in the bathwater can perform small miracles for those who believe themselves unloved or unlovable.

Herbs can also be used to strengthen the *chakras* – the body's spiritual centres defined in Eastern philosophy. The familiar kitchen basil (*Ocimum basilicum* – highly regarded in Ayurveda) is believed to reinforce the root, second and third *chakras*, while plants like lavender and elecampane are said to act on the crown *chakra*, which is associated with the pineal and pituitary glands. Using these types of herbs in conjunction with remedies for physical complaints can be very effective.

Modern science also has to accept that herbs can affect the mind and emotions in ways which we are only beginning to understand. There have been reports of aromatic chemicals from essential oils travelling through the

olfactory system to reach parts of the limbic centre in the brain – an area which in humans acts as a focus for emotions. Aromatherapy tends to be regarded in the UK as a massage-based technique, but purists in mainland Europe prefer to think of it – as the name implies – as a therapy associated with smells. Smelling certain oils can be stimulating and uplifting, while others have a more soothing and relaxing effect. Using oils in diffusers to scent rooms or adding a few drops to bath water are easy ways to influence the emotions. Oils from many of the herbs detailed in this book are especially useful and include chamomile, lavender, marjoram, melissa (lemon balm) and neroli (bitter orange).

Among the West's favourite remedies for emotional problems are the Bach Flower Remedies – discovered by Dr Edward Bach in the 1930s and used since then for soothing worries, fears and ill temper. The remedies are essentially the dew collected from particular plants preserved with brandy and seem to contain some invisible energy from the plant. They should be further diluted in water before being taken in drop doses. By this stage the remedies are in homoeopathic dilution and many orthodox herbalists are sceptical of their action. However, Bach Flower Remedies can be extremely helpful for a great many people and are worth trying.

the **Bach** flower **remedies**

Remedy	Dr Bach's suggested use
Agrimony	For those who suffer mental torture behind a "brave face"
Aspen	For vague fears of an unknown origin
Beech	For critical intolerance of others
Centaury	For the weak-willed
Cerato	For those who doubt their own judgement and seek advice of others
Cherry Plum	For fears of mental collapse
Chestnut Bud	For a refusal to learn from past mistakes
Chicory	For possessiveness and selfishness
Clematis	For the inattentive and dreamy escapist
Crab Apple	A cleansing remedy for those who feel unclean or ashamed
Elm	For those temporarily overcome by feelings of inadequacy
Gentian	For the despondent and easily discouraged
Gorse	For hopelessness and despair
Heather	For the self-centred obsessed with their own troubles
Holly	For those who are jealous, angry or feel hatred for others
Honeysuckle	For home sickness and nostalgia
Hornbeam	For "Monday morning feelings" and procrastination
Impatiens	For the impatient
Larch	For those who lack confidence
Mimulus	For fear of known things
Mustard	For deep gloom and depression

Remedy	Dr Bach's suggested use
Oak	For those who struggle on against adversity
Olive	For complete exhaustion
Pine	For guilt feelings and self-blame
Red Chestnut	For excessive fear for others, especially loved ones
Rock Rose	For extreme terror
Rock Water	For the self-repressed who overwork and deny themselves any relaxation
Scleranthus	For uncertainty and indecision
Star of Bethlehem	For shock
Sweet Chestnut	For extreme anguish; the limit of endurance
Vervain	For tenseness, over-enthusiasm and over-effort
Vine	For the dominating and inflexible
Walnut	For protection at times of change such as the menopause or during other major lifestage transitions
Water Violet	For the proud and reserved
White Chestnut	For mental anguish and persistent nagging worries
Wild Oat	For uncertainty about which path to take; an aid to decision taking
Wild Rose	For the apathetic who lack ambition
Willow	For the resentful and bitter who are fond of saying "not fair"

Having chosen a suitable selection of remedies put four drops of each into a 10 ml dropper bottle and then fill this with spring water. Take drop doses of the remedy on the tongue as required.

Plants that can help with the nervous system

The following herbs can be helpful – refer to Part 2 for details of use:

Almond
Apricot
Borage
Butterbur
Californian poppy
Chamomile
Coffee
Hawthorn
Lavender
Leek
Lemon balm
Lettuce
Linden
Nutmeg
Oats
Passion flower
Rosemary
Siberian ginseng
Skullcap
St John's wort
Valerian
Vervain
Wood betony

Skin problems

Our skin stands between us and the outside world: it must be porous enough to let out unwanted moisture in the form of sweat, but prevent us from being sodden in a rain shower. It has to provide protection from micro-organisms and pollution and it needs to be sufficiently soft and supple to allow a full range of energetic motions.

In Ayurvedic medicine, skin diseases are classified in terms of the three humours: too much *pitta* (fire) causes the blood to over-heat and poison the skin; too much *vata* (wind) causes dryness and itching, while *kapha* (damp) skin problems are related to weeping or oozing sores. Treatment focuses on balancing the offending humour.

The traditional approach of Western herbal medicine is to consider skin problems as related to blood impurities or circulating toxins, using herbs described as "depuratives" and "alteratives" to cleanse the system. Herbs like burdock, stinging nettles or cleavers are common favourites, while folk traditions include the use of carrots, grapes and turnips. These sorts of cleansing herbs are often combined with others to stimulate the liver or digestion and thus also improve elimination of toxins – laxatives like yellow dock, for example. Circulatory stimulants can be added to encourage a healthy oxygen supply and improve the quality of the tissues.

Although Western herbalists tend to emphasise internal remedies, external creams and lotions also have their place, especially for dry and scaling skin problems. Marigold, elder flower and chickweed creams are widely used. Aloe vera – which features in Ayurvedic, traditional Chinese and Western herbal medicine – is another favourite. More recently evening primrose and borage oils with their high *gamma*-linolenic acid content have moved into pole position and are recommended both internally and externally for numerous skin conditions, although they are really best for chronic, scaling, atopic eczema where a metabolic problem may be contributing to the cause.

Acne

The characteristic pimples and blackheads of acne are all too familiar to teenagers. Inflamed sebaceous glands – at their most active during puberty – are at the heart of the problem. The concentration of sebaceous glands varies over the body, so acne patches tend to be localised on the face, back and chest, although larger sebaceous cysts are more likely to occur on the scalp and genitals.

The conventional herbal approach is to cut down on the foods which might encourage sebaceous gland activity. This means reducing intake of refined carbohydrates (typically sugar and white flour), fried foods and animal fats. Sweets and chocolates also tend to aggravate the condition – as does excessive intake of alcohol and sweet, sugary drinks. Herbalists generally also recommend the internal use of alteratives as well as immune-strengthening herbs – like echinacea – if there is extensive infection.

Externally, topical use of antiseptic herbs can combat any infection associated with the excess sebum blocking hair follicles and causing pus to accumulate: a traditional stand-by is to rub a garlic clove on to the acne pustule each night – an effective cure, but one that rarely proves popular with spotty teenagers. Washing in cabbage water is another rather unpleasant folk cure – it does work well, but slightly more accept-able is cabbage lotion made by pulping cabbage leaves and distilled witch hazel in a food processor. Use this to cleanse and astringe the face twice a day.

Rather less aromatic are remedies like diluted tea tree oil and marigold. Steaming the skin with a mixture of hot water and a few drops of essential oils – such as marigold, chamomile or lavender – makes a good deep-cleansing treatment, or use facial washes containing a little finely powdered oatmeal instead of soap.

In Chinese medicine the exact location of the acne pustules is significant: suggesting where in the body there may be excess heat, believed in traditional Chinese medicine to contribute to the problem. Spots around the mouth, for example, can imply an over-heated stomach, while those around the nose are associated with the lung. Relevant cooling herbs for these organs are then included in the prescribed mix.

Eczema

Eczema and dermatitis (which simply means inflammation of the skin) are both terms used to describe non-contagious inflammatory skin conditions. The skin is usually red and itching with a rash, or there may be spots which can resemble small blisters which "weep" – ooze clear fluid to form a crust. "Dry eczema" involves a thickening and drying of the skin and is often characterised by dry, flaky patches.

Allergies – to chemicals, metals or certain foods – are a common cause and in children milk intolerance (especially among those who have not been breast-fed) is often the culprit. Since human milk is an excellent source of *gamma*-linolenic acid (see page 184), the illness has more recently been regarded as a failure in GLA metabolism. Persuading children to drink soya milk instead is not always easy, although it can often improve the condition. Food allergy also has aspects of addiction and dependence and children can literally be hooked on milk so, when the food is withdrawn, they can become irritable and unpleasant – much to their parents' despair.

Other likely dietary culprits include wheat, eggs and fruits that are rich in salicylates (especially tomatoes, oranges, berry fruits, peppers and aubergines), or shellfish. Tension and anxiety can also be contributory factors, and eczema sufferers often find symptoms increase when they are worried or under additional work or family pressures.

Once the cause has been identified, treatment usually involves use of alteratives to cleanse the body of any toxins, and demulcent creams to soften and help repair skin damage. A tea containing burdock, dandelion and yellow dock can be helpful; eat plenty of turnips and carrots and try lotions containing almond oil and evening primrose oil with essential oils of lavender, marigold or chamomile. Chickweed cream can help to relieve itching, and borage juice used externally can also help cool and ease highly irritant flare-ups.

In the elderly, poor circulation related to weakened veins can lead to yet another type of eczema – varicose

eczema – which may be associated with a tendency to develop varicose ulcers. Here, circulatory stimulants like ginkgo, ginger and cinnamon can help.

If stress is a problem, add soothing teas of chamomile, lemon balm, skullcap or wood betony to the regime.

Psoriasis

Emotional stresses also play a significant role in psoriasis – an extremely common condition associated with the failure of skin cells to develop normally. It is characterised by itchy, dry skin covered in silvery scales that flake off to reveal inflamed, red areas. The knees, legs, elbows, forearms and scalp are most frequently affected.

There is usually a family tendency to the problem and in some cases it can be associated with arthritis. Psoriasis generally first appears in the late teens or 20s and can then become a life-long problem. It tends to come and go for no apparent cause and will often disappear completely in the summer in response to plenty of sunshine and sea-bathing.

Herbal treatment usually involves the same sort of cleansing skin herbs used for eczema, as well as relaxing nervines to combat the associated stress. Alcohol should be strictly avoided as it dilates the peripheral blood vessels and encourages skin cell production still further.

An ideal treatment for minor cases is to apply a cream made from cleavers to small psoriatic patches as soon as they appear. Repeat two or three times a day. For psoriasis affecting the scalp, try hair rinses of a standard rosemary infusion with 5 drops of cade oil (see page 61) added. Cade oil can also be added to baths or creams.

Urticaria and hives

Highly irritant weals which can suddenly appear on the skin are variously described as urticaria, hives or nettle rash. They are often associated with an allergic reaction to some substance – either something taken internally or with which there has been skin contact. In severe cases there is also swelling of the hands, face, arms, eyelids or throat and there may be painful joints or breathing problems which can require emergency treatment.

Some people are sensitive to shellfish, others blame strawberries. However, a reaction to strawberries can also suggest an intolerance of foods containing salicylates (chemicals occurring widely in fruits, vegetables and many common herbs as well as also forming the basis of aspirin – another common cause of urticaria). Other drugs, including some antibiotics, can have a similar effect, so always check with your doctor if skin rashes follow a new prescription.

In traditional Chinese theory, nettle rash, which can affect different parts of the body at different times, is often blamed on "wind" – one of numerous evils which can attack us. Herbs to strengthen the immune systems (the surface defence energy or *Wei Qi*) are thus recommended. Possibilities for home use include echinacea and shiitake mushrooms. A favourite in China is schizandra fruit (*Schisandra chinensis*). The Chinese name for the herb, *Wu Wei Zi*, means "five taste seed", as it supposedly incorporates all five of the classic Chinese tastes – sweet, sour, salty, pungent and bitter – and it is a good *yin* tonic, promoting body fluids, encouraging secretions and strengthening energy levels. It can be quite effective for many allergic skin conditions.

Contact irritants can also cause urticaria – stinging nettles themselves are an obvious culprit. Their hairs actually contain histamine, a chemical normally present in the body, but one that in excess can trigger the characteristic allergic response. Orthodox remedies are thus generally based on anti-histamines and will work quickly and effectively. Other possibilities include insect stings (including bee stings and bee products), cosmetics, perfumes and a large number of common garden plants such as hops, runner bean tendrils, borage, yarrow, chamomile and rue (*Ruta graveolens*).

Urticaria is usually self-limiting and will clear in a few hours, but herbal remedies can provide soothing relief: useful remedies include chickweed cream, borage juice, fresh plantain leaves, lemon juice, sage ointment and distilled witch hazel.

Assorted infections

The skin is always contaminated by a large number of micro-organisms which generally cause us few problems. Stress, exhaustion or a weak immune system usually gives them the opportunity they need.

Athlete's foot (*Tinea pedis*) is a very common fungal infection affecting the space between the toes and toenails. Depending on the infecting fungus it can either involve inflammation and itching or may simply result in scaling skin and general discomfort. Like all their species, the yeasts causing athlete's foot thrive in warm, damp places, so good, sensible foot care – making sure the toes are well dried after bathing and that shoes are comfortable – is important. Using creams based on anti-fungal herbs, such as tea tree, marigold and echinacea, can help.

Boils are very tender inflamed areas of skin containing pus, generally caused by a staphylococcal infection of a hair follicle or a break in the skin. A cluster of boils is known as a carbuncle. Boils are usually a sign of reduced resistance to infection – perhaps because of general debility, chronic illness, exhaustion or overwork. There could also be some deep-seated septic focus such as a dental abscess adding to the over-all toxicity. Frequent outbreaks of boils can suggest a more serious underlying cause – possibly diabetes or kidney disease. Unskilled lancing of boils can spread infection and is best avoided. Herbal treatment can include the use of poultices or drawing ointments accompanied by antiseptic creams or lotions to encourage the boil to discharge. Effective external options include slippery elm, chickweed, tea tree and echinacea, with herbs such as hemp agrimony, garlic or echinacea taken internally to boost the immune system and combat bacterial infections.

Cold sores are caused by the herpes simplex Type I virus, which is believed to be carried by around 50% of the adult population. The sores are always quite localised and take the form of tiny blisters which usually start with a tingling sensation and rapidly develop to inflamed, red areas generally occurring around the mouth. Once a person has been infected, the virus can remain dormant in the body for years, usually causing a recurrent outbreak of sores if the sufferer is at all run down or over-tired. Women sometimes find that cold sores will coincide with menstruation and they can often herald a cold or flu simply because both can occur when resistance is weakened by exhaustion. The virus is extremely contagious during the blistering stage and can spread in saliva or by contact, so it is important to avoid touching the cold sore and spreading the infection to other parts of the body. Cold sores are more of a nuisance than a serious health hazard: try applying tea tree, marigold or lavender oils or creams as soon as the initial tingling sensation starts.

Dandruff is simply rather larger than usual flakes of dead skin which in the normal course of events would be more discreetly replaced every 28 days or so. It can be associated with seborrheic eczema where over-production of sebum (the natural oil secretions which lubricate the skin and hair) leads to oily, yellow flakes and often sore red patches on the scalp. Dandruff is believed to be caused, in part, by a fungal infection (due to *Pityrosporum ovale*), although it is not contagious and seems to depend on an individual over-response to the fungus. Wearing hats can make dandruff worse as the hot, damp environment they cause encourages fungal growth. Use of medicated shampoos can also worsen the condition because of the effect of detergents on scalp secretions and natural bacteria. Use the same sorts of cleansing remedies as for eczema (see page 171) and add infusions of rosemary leaves, chamomile flowers or stinging

nettle roots to hair rinses to improve scalp quality. Use gentle, soap-based shampoos rather than detergents.

Head lice epidemics are commonplace in schools. Lice are tiny brown insects about the size of a pinhead which lay six to eight eggs a day at the base of the hair shafts (usually at the nape of the neck or behind the ears). These hatch to produce white nymphs and discarded egg husks (nits). These live for about 20 days in an immature form – happily feeding on blood from the scalp – before pupating to the mature insect. Lice do not fly or jump, they simply walk from one head to another, which is easily achieved in the close confines of the classroom or playground. Tea tree is an ideal remedy: simply put a few drops of oil on a fine

Plants that can help with skin problems

The following herbs can be helpful – refer to Part 2 for details of use:

Almond	Cleavers	Marigold
Aloe	Common mallow	Marshmallow
Apple	Cucumber	Mustard
Apricot	Daisy	Oats
Arnica	Dandelion	Pineapple
Bilberry	Echinacea	Potato
Birch	Elder	Purple loosestrife
Bitter orange	Evening primrose	Slippery elm
Borage	Feverfew	St John's wort
Burdock	Fig	Stinging nettle
Cabbage	Golden seal	Strawberries
Carrot	Greater celandine	Tea
Chamomile	Herb Robert	Tea tree
Chickweed	Horseradish	Toadflax
Chili	Isphagula	Tomato
Cinnamon	Jack-by-the-hedge	Turnip
	Juniper	Walnut
	Lavender	Watercress
	Leek	Wheat
	Lemon	Yarrow
	Lettuce	Yellow dock

comb and comb the child's hair thoroughly night and morning, or add 10-20 drops of tea tree to 500 ml of hot water and use as a final hair rinse.

Warts are benign lumps in the skin caused by a virus which makes the cells multiply abnormally quickly. Common warts are usually found on the hands, knees and face and are mildly contagious, spreading as the virus comes into contact with damaged skin or when flakes from the wart touch other moist skin areas. Although they can be unsightly and a nuisance, these sorts of warts are usually quite harmless and most will disappear of their own accord. Useful herbal remedies include the sap of both greater celandine and dandelion, which can be squeezed onto warts each day until they disappear. The common garden weed, wood spurge (*Euphorbia amygdaloides*), is also known in some country districts as wart weed from the tradition of using its juice in a similar way. Professional help is needed for warts which appear to erupt on the site of moles or which start to bleed or change colour.

Verrucas are plantar warts that occur on the sole of the feet. Because they are always being walked on, the small growths can become painful and are often covered by thickened areas of skin or calluses. Readily available ring plasters and callous pads can provide some relief. The constant pressure also makes these warts grow inwardly rather than erupting outwards as with common warts; persistent cases usually need treatment from a chiropodist, although tea tree creams can help.

Urinary problems

Western medicine tends to regard the kidneys as mainly involved in water metabolism, although Ayurvedic medicine sees the kidneys as also influencing the nervous system and reproductive organs. In Chinese medicine, the kidney is believed to control the vital essence or *Jing* (see page 9) which affects both creative and sexual energies. The Chinese believe that if kidney energy is strong, an individual will show "determination" – be enthusiastic, clear thinking, vigorous and make "wise counsellors". Weak kidney energy leads to poor memory, few ambitions, low spirits or depression. In traditional Chinese medicine, the kidneys are associated with hearing and hair – it is a good sign when a baby is born with lots of hair as this indicates strong kidney *Qi* and *Jing*. Traditional Chinese medicine also links the kidneys with the emotion fear and maintains that they can be damaged by over-anxiety.

Persistent urinary problems can be seen as a weakness in kidney energy, so adding warming kidney tonics such as cinnamon to the urinary antiseptics and diuretics is often helpful.

Cystitis

Cystitis – literally inflammation of the bladder – is one of the most common "chronic" conditions affecting women. It is generally caused by infections ascending through the urethra – the tube that links the bladder to the outside world – to affect the bladder lining, so tends to be more common in women as their urethras are much shorter than men's: around 3.5 cm compared with about 20 cm. The symptoms will be familiar to many: a burning sensation on passing urine, a frequent need to do so and a dull ache in the lower abdomen.

Like all opportunist infections the bacteria which cause cystitis tend to get out of control when the sufferer is run down, so the problem often occurs when we are tired, overworked or under additional emotional stress. For many women cystitis follows sexual intercourse with monotonous regularity, leading to a reluctance to make love that can put considerable strain on a relationship.

Washing the area between urethra and anus (the perineum) after each bowel motion can help reduce the risk of counter infection, as can emptying the bladder within 10 or 15 minutes of intercourse and again washing the area. Bacteria thrive in warm, damp conditions so wearing loose panties, preferably cotton, and stockings instead of tights can help to keep the area around the urethra cool. Maintaining a more alkaline urine also discourages the bacteria, so opt for a more vegetarian diet, limiting meat intake and avoiding acidic foods like rhubarb, oranges and pickles.

Western herbal medicine has a wide range of herbs which modern science classifies as "urinary antiseptics" – usually herbs which include some chemical or other which is not broken down in the body and is excreted in the urine, thus producing a sort of internal disinfectant. Typical is cowberry or red whortleberry which has been found to contain 7% arbutin – a potent urinary antiseptic – in its leaves. Recent work in the USA has focused on the cranberry, a close relative of the cowberry. One study showed that clinical improvement was reported by 73% of cystitis sufferers given 480 ml of cranberry juice a day for 21 days.

Herbal remedies for cystitis also include diuretics, designed to flush out any toxins or infecting bacteria: buchu is one of the most useful as it is an antiseptic, diuretic and also warms the kidneys. Parsley is another good diuretic and, as with other herbs that "rob the soil", it is rich in minerals and vitamins so is useful in debilitated conditions: very large quantities of parsley, especially the seeds, are contraindicated in pregnancy as the herb may act as a uterine stimulant. Other useful diuretics likely to be found in the household medicine chest include agrimony, celery seed, leeks, pineapple juice, dandelion leaves and white deadnettle – all can be helpful for cystitis.

Astringents and wound herbs like agrimony, yarrow, purple loosestrife and shepherd's purse can also be useful in severe cases where there is blood in the urine. Echinacea is effective at combating kidney and urinary infections, so adding three 200 mg capsules, three times a day, to the therapeutic regime in acute cases can bring rapid improvement.

Prostate problems

Many men from their middle 40s onwards suffer from enlargement of the prostate gland. This sex gland sits beneath the bladder, surrounding the urethra, and contributes an alkaline fluid to the semen. As it enlarges it constricts the urethra, leading to hesitation in flow, dribbling, increased frequency of need to urinate and eventually retention of urine which can become a clinical emergency. Professional diagnosis is always needed

because of the possibility of prostate cancer – a common condition in older men but one which has a good five-year survival rate.

Prostate enlargement often seems to accompany retirement when a previously active man takes to the sedentary life with little exercise or energy. In Ayurvedic medicine prostate enlargement is also associated with diminished sexual activity – something which older men need not forsake and which can help to maintain kidney energy as well as keep the prostate gland healthy.

Herbal treatment tends to focus on energy-giving herbs, especially Siberian ginseng, and soothing diuretics, like white deadnettle. One very specific remedy is saw palmetto (*Serenoa repens*), which has been shown to prevent the conversion of the male hormone testosterone into dihydrotestosterone – a chemical now blamed for the excessive cell multiplication which leads to the enlargement of the prostate. In trials involving 110 prostate patients, saw palmetto reduced the incidence of night-time urination by 45% and significantly improved the urine flow for the majority of the sufferers. The dosage used in the trial was equivalent to 10 g of the berries twice a day – an extremely high dose – although herbalists often find much lower doses bring about a similar improvement.

At any age the prostate gland may also become infected, leading to prostatitis – an inflammation which can have cystitis-like symptoms and is similarly treated with urinary antiseptics, diuretics and soothing anti-inflammatories. Saw palmetto berries can also be helpful in these cases.

Plants that can help with the urinary system

The following herbs can be helpful – refer to Part 2 for details of use:

Agrimony
Asparagus
Bilberry
Bitter orange
Buchu
Carrot
Celery
Dandelion
Echinacea
Ginkgo
Juniper
Leek
Olive
Pineapple
Purple loosestrife
Self-heal
Shepherd's purse
Strawberries
Tomato
White deadnettle
Yarrow

Women's *ailments*

For centuries women had little other than herbs to sustain them through difficult periods, pregnancy and childbirth: the country names of many of our garden and wildflower healers remind us of the fact – lady's mantle, motherwort, mother's heart, milk thistle, maiden wort, lady's tresses and many more.

Steroidal compounds have been identified in many of these plants, explaining their potent effect on hormones and the menstrual cycle. Chaste-tree berries stimulate the pituitary gland to produce a variety of sex hormones involved in ovulation, while sage contains oestrogen-like compounds which explain its traditional use in drying up breast milk when weaning a baby and in reducing night sweats and hot flushes at the menopause.

Herbs can, however, do much more than simply provide an alternative to orthodox emphasis on hormones. Ayurvedic medicine stresses the importance of sexual energy in maintaining health and vitality and offers an impressive variety of herbs designed to help. In Ayurveda sexual energy is often equated with the creative energy used to improve mental or spiritual effort, so using herbs like basil (*Ocimum basilicum*) can be helpful.

Menstrual and reproductive disorders are many and varied and any change in blood flow or sudden irregularity can indicate problems which really need professional help. Self-diagnosis is not to be recommended – but for those commonplace and largely self-limiting monthly problems, herbs can provide a safe and gentle solution.

Pre-menstrual syndrome

Bloating, breast tenderness, irritability, anger, clumsiness, inability to concentrate… the symptoms of premenstrual syndrome (PMS) are many and varied. The problem can be explained in terms of falling progesterone levels and an orthodox approach thus tends to concentrate on hormone treatments – or use of chaste-tree berries (often given in tincture form, up to 20 drops each morning) as a herbal alternative. Dietary imbalance and candidiasis can also play a part and there is some evidence that cutting out artificial stimulants (themselves a possible stressor on the system) such as caffeine and theobromine in coffee, tea or chocolate can help. PMS has also been linked to various nutritional deficiencies and supplements – notably Vitamin B_6 and evening primrose oil – are often successfully used to relieve symptoms.

Herbal medicine can, however, offer a more holistic approach. In traditional Chinese medicine, premenstrual syndrome is seen as an energy imbalance often related to liver *Qi* (energy) congestion with symptoms of abdominal bloating, menstrual irregularities and period pain leading to a craving for sweet foods – a common PMS symptom – diarrhoea or constipation and fluid retention. Chinese remedies for PMS thus focus on energising and tonifying the liver using herbs like *Dang Gui* (see page 164). The Chinese consider that premenstrual breast distension is associated with rising *Qi*, so they add various bitter orange extracts to the mix to combat this trend. Taking 10 drops of bitter orange tincture in water three to four times a day can certainly help to ease these sorts of symptoms. Parsley tea is a popular

remedy for pre-menstrual fluid retention.

Women's monthly cycles have often been associated with the moon, with menstruation traditionally occurring at the time of the new moon and ovulation at the full. Some suggest that this natural rhythm is still followed by women whose main interests lie within the home, while for those more involved with external activities, menstruation coincides with the full moon instead. One way of regulating the menstrual cycle is to sleep with the curtains open, or a dull light glowing, at the time of a full moon and ensure complete darkness at the new moon.

A more recent remedy for menstrual problems has been evening primrose oil – now extensively and expensively marketed in numerous combinations to suit every stage of a woman's reproductive life. The *gamma*-linolenic acid it contains is believed to help with production of certain prostaglandins – hormone-like substances that can act as chemical messengers and also cause uterine contractions. GLA is contained in borage seed oil (often sold as starflower oil), but most women are able to produce it themselves in a normal metabolic process starting from *cis*-linoleic acid found in leafy plants and seed oils. For those on a tight budget a daily teaspoonful of good-quality walnut or safflower oil can make an adequate alternative to shrink-wrapped supplements.

Period pain

Herbalists tend to divide period pain into:
• Congestive pain, which builds up shortly before the period starts. It is associated with blood stagnation and blood congestion and can involve bloating and fluid retention. This sort of pain eases once the period has begun; and

• Spasmodic pain, due to uterine cramps which start once flow has begun and can be linked to a prostaglandin imbalance and emotional tension.

Relaxing anti-cramping remedies like chamomile, St John's wort or black haw bark (*Viburnum prunifolium*) are used for the spasmodic sort of pain, whereas more stimulating, hormonal or tonifying herbs like white deadnettle, raspberry leaf, rosemary, *Dang Gui* or chaste-tree can be helpful for the congestive variety.

Period pain can often be eased by exercise: rather than curling up with a hot water bottle and feeling miserable, try a brisk walk in the fresh air. Regular sexual intercourse – especially just before menstruation starts – can also help to reduce period pain, while some argue that intercourse during the period is the best way of easing cramps – although there are numerous cultural taboos arguing against intercourse at such times.

Period pain can also – as with PMS – be associated with liver stagnation and so can be exacerbated by alcohol and highly processed foods.

Heavy periods

Heavy periods can sometimes indicate some major underlying problems – such as fibroids or endometriosis – but often they have no apparent cause and are more of an irritant than anything else. Modern medicine tends to respond to complaints of heavy periods with suggestions for hysterectomies which, sadly, many women accept as the only solution. Hysterectomy is something to be avoided if at all possible. In Ayurvedic theory the various energy centres of the body, the *chakras*, start with the root

chakra which in women is found at the womb. Removing this organ thus tends to leave women feeling "rootless" and can lead to emotional disturbances.

Menstrual "heaviness" is also relative: some women always have heavy periods and to them this is normal; others find periods get heavier with age and start to worry. The main thing is to seek professional advice if the pattern of flow changes significantly, but not to be persuaded into unnecessary treatments.

Useful herbs to combat excessive flow include shepherd's purse (also known as mother's hearts), marigold, herb Robert, hawthorn and white deadnettle.

Vaginal thrush

Recurrent vaginal thrush often indicates an underlying problem with candidiasis or food intolerance, as the immune system is constantly under stress and unable to combat opportunist bugs like *Candida albicans*. Taking echinacea or garlic can help counter the infection and strengthen the immune system, while anti-fungal creams such as tea tree or marigold can help to give symptomatic relief.

Tea tree has become extremely popular in recent years with commercially made pessaries containing the oil now sold in many health-food shops. Unlike most essential oils, tea tree does not irritate the mucous membranes and most people can tolerate it used neat instead of diluted in a vegetable carrier oil.

A simple application technique is to use a tampon: push it slightly out of the tube and moisten the top with water. Then add 3 drops of tea tree oil to the exposed moist top and insert it in the vagina. Leave for three to fours hours and repeat twice a day.

Pregnancy and childbirth

Herbs have a long tradition of use for easing the pains of childbirth and the ills of pregnancy: for generations of women they were the only available remedies and much folklore – as well as hard scientific evidence – testifies to their efficacy. Today few women in the West have the opportunity to use herbs in this way: childbirth has become a much more orderly and monitored affair.

Using herbs in pregnancy also needs caution: many contain chemicals that will cross the placental barrier, so it is unwise to take any remedies in the first three months unless you really have to. The list of herbs to be avoided in pregnancy is already long and growing as potential new hazards are identified and, frequently, exaggerated (see Cautions, page 12, for details of those to avoid). Many herbs are, however, perfectly safe to use and even most of those which should be avoided in high, regular doses are fine in moderation.

Morning sickness, which affects many pregnant women in the first three months is generally, fortunately, confined to a few minutes on rising, although with some sufferers it can last all day and extend through much of the nine months. Researchers have found that ginger is extremely effective even in these very severe cases. Up to 1 g per dose has been used quite safely in hospital trials. Other herbs that can help include fennel, lemon balm, bitter orange, chamomile and peppermint. These are best kept as tinctures in dropper bottles on the bedside table and used before rising. Alternatively, leave a Thermos flask of a suitable herbal infusion beside the bed at night so that the mix is ready to take before rising next morning. Try different remedies as need be – morning sickness may respond well to a particular remedy on one occasion but not on another, so keep plenty of alternatives nearby.

Heartburn in pregnancy can be safely treated with slippery elm or marshmallow, while for *constipation* (often exacerbated by the use of supplementary iron tablets) stay with the gentler remedies – isphaghula, yellow dock or dandelion root.

Childbirth: Raspberry leaf has long been used to strengthen the womb ready for childbirth: it helps to tonify the uterus and aid contractions, but should be taken only in the last eight weeks of pregnancy. During labour many teas have traditionally been used to help relaxation, soothe pain and encourage contractions. In the modern labour ward sipping a home-brewed cup of herbal tea is not always possible, but they can certainly be used in the early stages of labour or where midwives are sympathetic. Traditional mixtures include wood betony and chamomile, with rose petal, raspberry leaf and clove in the later stages. Massaging the abdomen with well-diluted clove or sage oils can also help. To speed recovery from the birth itself, homoeopathic Arnica 6X tablets taken every 15-30 minutes for a few hours will help repair stressed tissues.

Breast-feeding problems: Sore nipples in breast-feeding are commonplace: the cause is often poor positioning of the baby, who should suck at the whole areola (the dark area around the nipple) rather than just holding on to the nipple itself. Marigold and chamomile creams can help.

Many herbs, including fennel and vervain, also encourage milk flow. To dry up milk at weaning take sage tea.

Menopausal problems

For most women the menopause passes by with little more inconvenience than occasional hot flushes and night sweats. For others, it can be a time of major emotional upheaval, depression, weight gain and heavy bleeding.

Today, many of these symptoms may be treated by hormone replacement therapy which boosts oestrogen levels, although critics still have doubts about the long-term effects of such treatment. For some women (including those with a high risk of osteoporosis) HRT can be a preferred solution, but for those who want to complete this transition period in their lives as naturally as possible, then exercise, an increase in calcium intake and herbal remedies – to relieve the more troublesome symptoms and help the body to adjust to new levels of functionality – can be far better. A normally healthy lifestyle with good diet, a happy and fulfilled outlook and acceptable stress levels is also obviously important. Anyone who starts out being depressed, overworked or malnourished is unlikely to pass through the menopause without trauma.

Traditional Chinese theory associated menopausal problems with a run-down in the kidney's vital energy and using kidney tonics to ease symptoms can be extremely effective. Herbs like cinnamon and buchu which have a tonic effect on the kidneys can be worth trying and there are a number of specialist Chinese tonic herbs (such as *He Shou Wu* – *Polygonum multiflorum*) which are now

appearing in over-the-counter menopausal products.

Many herbs can be used to ease the more troublesome menopausal symptoms – sage and golden seal can help with hot flushes, chaste-tree will regulate hormone production, while the emotional ups and downs can be soothed with skullcap, borage, St John's wort or lemon balm. Hawthorn is useful for easing menopausal palpitations, while vaginal dryness can often be helped with creams containing Vitamin E and marigold.

Plants that can help with women's ailments

The following herbs can be helpful – refer to Part 2 for details of use:

Borage
Celery
Chaste-tree
Evening primrose
Fennel
Golden seal
Hawthorn
Marigold
Sage
Shepherd's purse
Skullcap
Stinging nettle
Thyme
Vervain
White deadnettle
Witch hazel

Wound herbs

Herbs have been used for centuries for all sorts of injuries and wounds. Their very names remind us of the fact: yarrow's botanical name (*Achillea*) comes from Achilles, who reputedly used it before the gates of Troy to heal his fellow Greeks. In some cultures a warlike nature tended to dominate views of herbs: the Maori of New Zealand, for example, were always fighting each other and the vast majority of their traditional remedies involve poultices and compresses to heal the injured.

Herbs are still ideal for all sorts of minor cuts, grazes and burns: the choice is wide, so even when you are far from home there is generally a suitably styptic healer close at hand.

Burns and sunburn

Burns are potential medical emergencies and only the most minor should be treated at home. Any burn more than about 5 cm across should be seen by a doctor as soon as possible. For less severe injuries running cold water over the affected area or using an ice pack (or packet of frozen peas) will cool it down and ease the immediate pain. Keeping the injury cool for two or three hours can often help significantly.

Useful topical herbs for burns include aloe vera, bilberry, powdered coffee beans, lavender, pot marigold, raw potato, chickweed, white deadnettle, butterbur and St John's wort.

Given the publicity in recent years of the risks of skin cancer from sunbathing in our ozone-depleted environment, one would imagine that we would all remain well protected under sun hats and long-sleeved shirts. However, perhaps because the sun's rays are more penetrative in our polluted atmosphere, sunburn seems ever more commonplace. St John's wort oil is a useful standby for emergencies – add 2 ml of lavender oil to 18 ml of St John's wort oil in a 20 ml bottle and include it in the holiday first-aid kit.

Cuts and grazes

Herbal alternatives to the usual mixture of orthodox antiseptic creams which fill the average domestic first-aid box are now readily available. Always bathe cuts and grazes by either rinsing the wound under running water or using cotton wool soaked in warm water or an infusion of antiseptic herbs, taking care to wipe from centre to edge of the graze to clear any grime. Pressing a clean tissue or gauze pad over the injury for a few minutes will also stop bleeding. Finally, apply antiseptic creams – marigold (calendula), echinacea, St John's wort or tea tree creams are all suitable and can be used on open wounds.

Aloe vera creams can also be used on grazes and various combinations containing St John's wort are commercially available. In the past, comfrey was generally recommended to encourage healing; however, given recent concerns over the toxic alkaloids it contains (see page 142), many now advise against its being used on open wounds.

The list of wound herbs is long and impressive – if far from home look for agrimony, bear's breech, chickweed, coltsfoot, creeping Jenny, hemp agrimony, herb Robert, Jack-by-the-hedge, marsh woundwort, marshmallow, self-heal, shepherd's purse or yarrow.

Insect bites and stings

For most people insect bites and stings in temperate zones lead to little more than local irritation which eases in a few days. However, for an unfortunate minority stings lead to severe allergic reactions which can range from weeping and persistent dermatitis to anaphylactic shock characterised by dizziness, sickness, breathing problems and marked swelling of the affected area. When severe, this can be fatal. Immediate emergency medical treatment is vital in such cases.

Bees will sting only if they or their hives are attacked, as the hooked barb on the sting cannot be withdrawn and the insect dies defending itself. Wasps have a straight sting and can, rather unpleasantly, repeatedly attack their victims. Bee stings are acidic and in traditional first aid were treated with blue-bag (an alkaline starch used in laundry) or bicarbonate of soda, while alkaline wasp stings were soothed by vinegar. Both, however, respond well to slices of onion or leek.

To soothe irritant mosquito and gnat bites try rubbing them with fresh common plantain leaves, aloe vera sap or lemon balm leaves, lemon juice, slices of cucumber or tomato, or use infusions or ointments containing sage. If bites become infected, echinacea or tea tree cream can be helpful.

Keeping the insects away is another way of tackling the problem and several herbal oils will help here: tea tree and lemon balm are ideal sprinkled on clothing; at barbecues or when sitting out of doors, try burning citronella (*Cymbopogon nardus*) candles.

<table>
<tr><td colspan="3">**Plants that can help with minor injuries**</td></tr>
</table>

	Cucumber	Sage
The following herbs can be helpful – refer to Part 2 for details of use:	Daisy	Self-heal
	Echinacea	Shepherd's purse
	Golden seal	Slippery elm
	Herb Robert	St John's wort
Agrimony	Jack-by-the-hedge	Strawberries
Aloe	Leek	Tea
Arnica	Lemon balm	Tea tree
Bear's breech	Marigold	Thyme
Beetroot	Marsh woundwort	Toadflax
Bilberry	Olive	Tomato
Butterbur	Onion	White deadnettle
Chamomile	Pineapple	Witch hazel
Chickweed	Plantain	Wood avens
Coffee	Potato	Yarrow
Comfrey	Purple loosestrife	
Creeping Jenny	Raspberry	

Herbs for *babies* *and* *children*

Many herbs are quite safe for children – although unfortunately, the taste is often far from pleasant and administering the remedy can prove a problem. Giving babies weak infusions of soothing herbs, such as chamomile or linden, by bottle from a very early age can encourage acceptance of herby flavours, while dosing breast-fed babies can often be best achieved by the mother taking the herbal remedy herself, as many of the active ingredients will then pass into the breast milk. This is an especially neat solution for colic and wind remedies (see below), which can thus be dispensed precisely at feeding time.

Toddlers can be dosed with teaspoons of honey containing herb powders or drops of tinctures, while capsules are ideal and tasteless just as soon as children are old enough to swallow them. Tinctures (neat or dilute, depending on age) given in drop doses on the tongue can also be quite accept-able – the process can even be made into a game that can override the unpleasantness of the taste.

Taste is held to be more significant in some cultures than in others: Ayurvedic medicine, for example, divides tastes into six categories: sweet, sour, salty, pungent, bitter and astringent. A child's healthy growth depends on a good balance of tastes, and special sweets and pills are sold which combine all six tastes with which parents can dose their children.

Herbal dosages need, of course, to be reduced for children. Much depends on the child's size but a general guide is given in this table.

Children's dosages

Age	Dose
0-1 year	5% of adult dose
1-2 years	10% of adult dose
3-4 years	20% of adult dose
5-6 years	30% of adult dose
7-8 years	40% of adult dose
9-10 years	50% of adult dose
11-12 years	60% of adult dose
13-14 years	80% of adult dose
15-plus	100% of adult dose

In many childhood illnesses herbs can help to calm over-excitement, ease tension and encourage sleep – which will all significantly aid the healing process. Chamomile, linden and lemon balm are ideal taken in infusions and sweetened with honey. If over-excitement leads to nervous exhaustion then give oatmeal porridge or oatcakes, along with vervain and wood betony infusions. Older children can also be safely given Californian poppy for sleeplessness, while some preparations containing passion flower can also be suitable.

Children also suffer the same

complaints as their elders, so reduced doses of many of the remedies suggested for coughs, constipation and stomach upsets will generally be suitable. For infections, low doses of echinacea are quite safe. Children can develop dramatically high fevers with the temperature reaching 39°C (102°F) or more. Raising the body temperature is part of the normal defence mechanism to combat invading organisms and is not generally a problem. However, if the temperature rises above 39°C (102°F) for more than 24 hours, professional help is advisable. For milder cases herbal remedies containing elder flower, yarrow and linden can be helpful. Especially suitable for children is catmint (*Nepeta cataria*), which can easily be grown in gardens and makes an ideal tea for feverish conditions and minor stomach upsets.

Catarrhal problems

Persistent catarrh in childhood is often associated with milk allergy, so try switching to soya milk instead of cow's. Soya is a good source of calcium and other minerals, so completely eliminating dairy products from a child's diet is unlikely to cause any deficiencies – although if possible you should avoid the genetically modified soya products now coming on to the market. Soya-based yoghurts and desserts which can be suitable for children are also now commercially available. Gentle herbs for catarrhal conditions include elder flower and ribwort plantain. Eliminating milk can also be helpful in many cases of glue ear (*secretory otitis media*, see page 162).

Colic

This is a severe abdominal pain which tends to come in waves a few seconds or minutes apart. In adults it can be due to an obstruction in the intestine or simply to constipation and can need professional treatment. In babies, colic is usually caused by air becoming trapped in the intestines and is generally associated with feeding difficulties – or a failure to "wind" the infant properly after it has finished sucking. Colicky babies often remain so for the first three months of life, which can be extremely wearing on the parents as the child's only reaction to the pain it feels is to cry – loudly. Traditional gripe water is, of course, a herbal remedy usually based on dill extracts. Alternatively, use weak infusions of fennel or dill. Another suitable option for colic is homoeopathic chamomile (Chamomilla 3X), which is available in drops or pilules.

Cradle cap

A dandruff-like condition that affects young babies and usually starts with scurf on the head followed by the development of yellow, crusted scaly patches. These can spread over the whole head or simply be confined to particular areas. The condition is quite harmless and may be related to overactivity of the sebaceous glands in the scalp, possibly caused by the mother's hormones. A simple remedy is to rub olive or wheatgerm oil gently into the baby's scalp, allow it to soak well in and then wash the flakes away; infused marigold or heartsease (*Viola tricolor*) oils and creams can also be safely used.

Digestive upsets

Persistent bilious attacks are common with some children and are often identified as a type of migraine. Eliminating the sort of foods that adult migraine sufferers commonly find trigger attacks (such as cheese and chocolate) can help. The soothing carminatives – lemon balm, chamomile, fennel – are also worth trying. Childhood constipation needs to be treated with gentle remedies and definitely not the sort of stimulating laxatives that adults may favour (avoid senna and other anthraquinone-containing herbs). Isphaghula seeds are a good bulking laxative. One way to get children to take them is to disguise them with breakfast cereal: put the seeds in the bowl, then add the cereal and milk. The mucilaginous, swollen seeds will generally be swallowed with the soggy cornflakes without too many complaints. Commercial "flavoured" isphaghula remedies are available for children. Yellow dock or liquorice can also be suitable – or you can opt for the many laxative foods such as apples, pears or dried apricots.

Hyperactivity

Food allergies can also account for many cases of hyperactivity – colourants like tartrazine (E102) and sunset yellow (E110) are particularly suspect. Hyperactivity is explained in Chinese medicine in terms of liver *Qi* disharmonies or flaring of liver fire, so suitable liver herbs like vervain, agrimony or self-heal can be used in combination with gentle sedatives like chamomile, lemon balm, Californian poppy or skullcap.

Nappy rash

Sore, red bottoms seem to develop in
some children no matter how carefully
the mother changes and dries the little
one. It is important to keep the affected
area as dry as possible (even by blowing
with a hair dryer set to the cool setting).
It is better to use ointments than creams,
as they form a protective barrier for the
skin whereas creams tend to soak in and
soften. Marigold, chamomile or comfrey
ointment can be helpful and safe to use,
as can aloe vera gel. Bacteria in the faeces
can react with urine to produce
ammonia and this can encourage fungal
infections similar to thrush to develop. If
this occurs, use ointments containing
marigold or tea tree.

Teething

Cutting those first teeth can start from
around six months and can be a gruelling
time for all members of the family.
Homoeopathic Chamomilla 3X remedies
can be very soothing; some babies will
take weak chamomile tea from a bottle
or it can be added to bathwater to
encourage more restful nights.

Plants that can be helpful for children

*The following herbs can be helpful –
refer to Part 2 for details of use:*

Agrimony
Almond
Aloe
Apple
Californian poppy
Chamomile
Cloves
Creeping Jenny
Echinacea
Ginger
Lemon balm
Lettuce
Liquorice
Olive
Peppermint
Pilewort
Raspberry
Self-heal
Shepherd's purse
Tea tree
Watercress
White deadnettle
Witch hazel
Wood avens
Yarrow

gloss**ary**

Adaptagen a substance that helps the body to adapt to a new strain or stress, supporting the immune system and initiating regeneration of tissues and fluids. Herbal adaptagens include Korean ginseng, Siberian ginseng, shiitake mushrooms and *gotu kola* (*Centella asiatica*).

Adrenal cortex part of the adrenal gland located above the kidneys, which produces several steroidal hormones.

Alkaloid active plant constituent containing nitrogen and which usually has a significant effect on bodily function.

Allergen any substance which triggers an allergic response.

Allopathy prevalent system of Western medicine which treats illness by prescribing substances to provoke an opposite condition from the disease – thus a fever is treated with temperature suppressants or an ache with pain-killers.

Alterative a substance which improves the function of various organs – notably those involved with the breakdown and excretion of waste products – to bring about a gradual change of state.

Amino acids the building blocks of proteins.

Amoebacidal kills amoeba.

Analgesic relieves pain.

Anaesthetic causes local or general loss of sensation.

Anaphrodisiac reduces sexual desire and excitement.

Anodyne allays pain.

Anthelmintic destroys or expels worms.

Antibiotic destroys or inhibits growth of micro-organisms such as bacteria and fungi.

Anti-bacterial destroys or inhibits the growth of bacteria.

Anti-fungal destroys or inhibits the growth of fungi.

Anti-inflammatory reduces inflammation.

Anti-microbial destroys or inhibits the growth of micro-organisms such as bacteria and fungi.

Anti-oxidant prevents or slows the natural deterioration of cells that occurs as they age due to oxidation.

Anti-rheumatic relieves the symptoms of rheumatism.

Antiseptic controls or prevents infection.

Antispasmodic reduces muscle spasm and tension.

Anti-tussive inhibits the cough reflex, helping to stop coughing.

Aperient a very mild laxative.

Aphrodisiac promotes sexual excitement.

Aril fleshy or hairy outgrowth of certain seeds.

Astringent used to describe a herb which will precipitate proteins from the surface of cells or membranes causing tissues to contract and tighten; forms a protective coating and stops bleeding and discharges.

Atherosclerosis build-up of fatty deposits in the blood vessels leading to narrowing and hardening and associated with heart disease and strokes.

Bach Flower Remedies extracts of flowers collected as dew and preserved in brandy, discovered by Dr Edward Bach in the 1930s and widely used to treat emotional upsets and disturbances (see page 169 for details of Dr Bach's 38 healers).

Bactericidal kills bacteria.

Beta-carotene an orange-yellow plant pigment which is converted in the body into vitamin A.

Biennial a plant which lives for two years.

Bile thick, bitter fluid secreted by the liver and stored in the gall bladder which aids the digestion of fats.

Bitter stimulates secretion of digestive juices.

Blood clotting the process by which the proteins in blood are changed from a liquid to a solid by an enzyme, in order to check bleeding.

Blood sugar levels of glucose in the blood.

Bronchial relating to the air passages of the lungs.

Bulk laxative increases the volume of faeces producing larger, softer stools.

Capillary permeability the exchange of carbon dioxide, oxygen, salts and water between the blood in capillaries and tissues.

Carcinogenic causes cancer.

Carminative expels gas from the stomach and intestines to relieve flatulence, digestive colic and gastric discomfort.

Cathartic a strong, purging laxative.

Cerebral circulation blood supply to the brain.

Chakra a Buddhist concept of human energy centres which can be visualised as blazing whirlpools of light in the energy field surrounding the body and between which energy flows. There are seven *chakras*, each connected with a different part of the body: the "root" or "basic" *chakra* at the base of the spine, the "spleen" *chakra* over the spleen, the "navel" *chakra* at the solar plexus, the "heart" *chakra* over the heart, the "throat" *chakra* at the front of the throat, the "brow" *chakra* in the space between the eyebrows and the "crown" or "coronal" *chakra* on the top of the head.

Choleric one of the Galenical temperaments associated with yellow bile, heat and dryness.

Cholesterol fat-like material present in the blood and most tissues which is an important constituent of cell membranes, steroidal hormones and bile salts. Excess cholesterol has been blamed for the build-up of fatty deposits in the blood vessels seen in atherosclerosis.

Choleretic increases the secretion of bile by the liver.

Circulatory stimulant increases blood flow.

Cleansing herb a herb that improves the excretion of waste products from the body.

Cooling used to describe herbs that are often bitter or relaxing and will help to reduce internal heat and hyperactivity.

Coumarin active plant constituent which affects blood clotting.

Decongestant relieves congestion, usually nasal.

Demulcent softens and soothes damaged or inflamed surfaces, such as the gastric mucous membranes.

Depressant reduces nervous or functional activity.

Diaphoretic increases sweating.

Diuretic encourages urine flow.

Doctrine of Signatures a medieval theory which argued that plants contained clues to their medicinal properties in their appearance: yellow-flowered herbs, for example, were believed to be helpful for jaundice, while pilewort with its nodular roots was clearly ideal for treating haemorrhoids. Some of these interpretations were quite valid (pilewort *is* good for haemorrhoids and yellow-flowered dandelion makes a good liver herb); others, now largely forgotten, were less accurate. Similar beliefs are found in most cultures worldwide.

Emetic causes vomiting.

Emmenagogue restores or brings on menstruation.

Emollient softens and soothes the skin.

Essential fatty acids these are classified by chemical structure and the two groups most commonly found in supplements are known as *omega*-six and *omega*-three acids. The *omega*-six group includes arachidonic acid and *gamma*-linolenic acid (GLA), while the *omega*-three category includes linoleic acid, *alpha*-linolenic acid and two commonly found in fish oil – eicosapentanoeic acid (EPA) and docasahexaenic acid (DHA). In recent years these acids have been found to be of significant nutritional importance and lack of them is believed to contribute to a very wide range of common Western ills – including arthritis, skin diseases, menstrual and menopausal problems and heart disease. A number of acids can be metabolised in the body from linoleic acid but only when it is in its chemical *cis*-linoleic form. Commercially produced vegetable oils often convert this form into *trans*-linoleic acid in processing and this is less beneficial. *Gamma*-linolenic acid is found in evening primrose oil, borage oil and blackcurrant oil and these oils also contain substantial amounts of *cis*-linoleic acid. *Alpha*-linolenic acid is found in significant amounts in linseed, hemp seed and pumpkin seed oils

with less in walnut and soy bean oils.

Not all essential fatty acids are beneficial – erucic acid is believed to damage heart tissue, for example, and is found in high proportion in certain varieties of rape seed (and in trace amounts in some borage seed extracts).

The essential fatty acids are important in the production of prostaglandins. More than 50 of these have been identified and they have wide-ranging and important functions in the body. The PGE_1 series is particularly beneficial and these are often at low levels in people who are prone to allergies, depressives, alcoholics and diabetics. In the usual metabolic pathway *cis*-linoleic is converted to *gamma*-linolenic acid which in turn is made into *dihomogamma*-linolenic acid in the body which is then used to make PGE_1.

Essential oils volatile chemicals extracted from plants by such techniques as steam distillation; highly active and aromatic.

Expectorant enhances the secretion of sputum from the respiratory tract so that it is easier to cough up.

Febrifuge reduces fever.

Flavonoids active plant constituents which improve the circulation and may also have diuretic, anti-inflammatory and antispasmodic effects.

Galactogogue promotes secretion of milk.

Galenical medicine traditional Western medicine practised throughout Europe until the 18th century and largely based on ancient Greek principles dating back to Hippocrates. The theory took its name from Galen, a Graeco-Roman physician, and regards human health and temperament as controlled by four bodily humours: phlegm, yellow bile, black bile and blood, giving rise to the temperaments: phlegmatic, choleric, melancholic and sanguine.

***Gamma*-linolenic acid** see **Essential fatty acids**.

Haemostatic stops bleeding.

Hormone a chemical substance produced in the body which can affect the way tissues

behave. Hormones can control sexual function and emotional and physical activity.

Humours substances associated with bodily states or temperaments in both Galenical and Ayurvedic medicine. The Galenical humours were blood, yellow bile, black bile and phlegm. Ayurvedic humours are *vata* (air), *pitta* (fire) and *kapha* (water).

Hyperacidity excessive digestive acid causing a burning sensation.

Hyperglycaemic increases blood sugar levels.

Hypertensive raises blood pressure.

Hypoglycaemic reduces blood sugar levels.

Hypotensive lowers blood pressure.

Labyrinth the inner ear

Laxative encourages bowel motions.

Lipids fat-like chemicals (such as cholesterol), present in most tissues and important structural materials for the body.

Lubricant reduces friction.

Melancholic one of the Galenical temperaments associated with black bile, cold and dryness.

Ménière's disease a disorder of the inner ear which leads to nausea, vertigo, tinnitus and deafness. The cause is largely unknown.

Menthol a volatile oil with a peppermint aroma extracted from various mints (including peppermint) which is carminative, locally anaesthetic, decongestant and antiseptic. Used in a number of herbal products for colds and indigestion.

Mucilage complex sugar molecules found in plants that are soft and slippery and provide protection for the mucous membranes and inflamed surfaces.

Nervine herb that affects the nervous system and which may be stimulating or sedating.

Peripheral circulation blood supply to the limbs, skin and muscles (including heart muscles).

Peristalsis waves of involuntary contractions in the digestive tract which move food and waste through the system.

Phlegm catarrhal-like secretion or sputum. In both Galenical and Oriental medicine phlegm is a more complex entity related to internal balance and sometimes associated with spleen deficiency.

Phlegmatic one of the Galenical temperaments associated with phlegm, cold and dampness.

Photosensitivity sensitivity to light.

Physiomedicalism system of medicine developed in 19th-century North America which focused on disease as a result of cold conditions.

Pineal gland a pea-shaped mass of tissue found in the brain, believed to have some function in sexual development and known to secrete the hormone melatonin.

Pituitary gland a major gland in the endocrine system controlling production of many vital hormones. Located at the base of the skull.

Prostaglandins hormone-like substances that have a wide range of functions in the body. They can act as chemical messengers and some also cause uterine contractions. Various series of prostaglandins are known, usually designated PGE_1, PGE_2, etc.

Pungent having an acrid smell and bitter flavour.

Purgative drastic laxative.

Pyrrolizidine alkaloids chemicals found in a number of plants (including comfrey, borage and coltsfoot) which in excess can be associated with liver damage, although many regard the research evidence for this as inconclusive.

Qi (ch'i) the body's vital energy as defined in Chinese medicine.

Relaxant relaxes tense and overactive nerves and tissues.

Rubefacient a substance which stimulates blood flow to the skin, causing local reddening.

Sanguine one of the Galenical temperaments associated with blood, heat and dampness. It was regarded in the Middle Ages as the ideal temperament.

Saponins active plant constituents similar to soap and producing a lather with water. They can irritate the mucous membranes of the digestive tract which, by reflex, has an expectorant action. Some saponins are chemically similar to steroidal hormones.

Sedative reduces anxiety and tension.

Simple a herb used as a remedy on its own.

Soporific induces drowsiness and sleep.

Stimulant increases activity.

Styptic stops external bleeding.

Systemic affecting the whole body.

Tannin active plant constituents which are astringent and combine with proteins. The term is derived from plants used in tanning leather.

Thyroid gland in the neck which controls metabolism and growth; it requires iodine for normal function.

Tincture liquid herbal extract made by soaking plant material in a mixture of alcohol and water.

Tisane an infusion.

Tonic restoring, nourishing and supporting for the entire body.

Tonifying having a tonic action: strengthening and restoring for the system.

Topical local administration of a herbal remedy.

Venous return the blood flow back to the lungs and heart from the body's extremities.

Volatile oils complex, often aromatic, substances with a low boiling point which rapidly evaporate in the air. The smells associated with different herbs and extracts are often due to such oils.

Vulnerary wound herb.

Warming a remedy which increases body temperature and encourages digestive function and circulation. Warming herbs are often spicy and pungent to taste.

Yang aspect of being equated with male energy – dry, hot, light, ascending.

Yin aspect of being equated with female energy – damp, cold, dark, descending.

consulting a herbalist

While over-the-counter herbal remedies can be helpful for a range of ailments, more serious problems need professional help. Approaches to herbal medicine vary considerably around the world. In the UK, primary health care is dominated by conventionally trained general practitioners whose attitudes to alternative or complementary therapies range from the sympathetic to the openly hostile: a few GPs may be trained in herbal or homoeopathic medicine or, if not, may be willing to refer patients to suitable practitioners but many more dismiss herbal medicine as "quackery". In France herbal practitioners or *phyto-therapists* are almost always trained doctors who have studied plant medicine at post-graduate level, while in Germany, alternative practitioners qualify as *heilpraktiker* and have comparable status to orthodox GPs.

In China, traditional herbal medicine is available in special hospitals as an alternative to Western medicine, while in Japan herbal remedies are available on the equivalent of the National Health Service. In certain other countries – including some states of the USA – it is illegal for anyone to prescribe herbal remedies or set themselves up as a herbal practitioner, although self medication with herbs is permitted. In others just about anyone – well trained or not – can set up in business as a medical herbalist and dispense all manner of inappropriate "cures".

Britain is probably unique within Europe in having a well-established and reputable system for training herbal practitioners who have not necessarily obtained any other medical qualifications. The National Institute of Medical Herbalists was founded in 1864 and members qualify by examination after four or five years of specialist study. Many overseas students also attend courses run by the School of Phytotherapy in the

UK in Sussex, and there are now two UK universities offering degree courses in herbal medicine. Members of the National Institute use the initials MNIMH or FNIMH after their names which gives the patient some guarantee that they are consulting a suitably trained practitioner.

The UK's other main professional herbal body is the General Council and Register of Herbalists, whose members use the initials MH. It has a rather different philosophical approach from that usually adopted by the NIMH practitioners with its members tending more towards homoeopathy: herbal tinctures are likely to be prescribed in drop doses rather than the teaspoonful generally favoured by NIMH members. A third, more recently formed organisation is the Register of Traditional Chinese Medicine, whose members largely use a combination of acupuncture and Chinese herbs.

Australia has a strong tradition of naturopathy, with practitioners likely to combine dietary advice, herbal medicines and aromatherapy. Trained herbalists are often members of the National Herbalists Association of Australia and use the initial MNHAA after their names; they are classified as Health Care Professionals by the Australian government and may practise privately or in association with more orthodox practitioners.

Herbal training in New Zealand is rather more fragmented, with a number of herb schools and no single recognised form of certification. There is, however, growing interest in using indigenous plants as alternatives to European herbs and several groups are extremely active in this area. A number of practitioners in both Australia and New Zealand are also members of the British National Institute of Medical Herbalists and – as in the UK – add MNIMH after their names.

In both the USA and Canada, herbal practice tends to be fragmented and legal controls can vary considerably between both states and provinces. Canadian groups include the Ontario Herbalists'

Association, Central Canadian Herbal Practitioners' Association, La Guilde des Herboristes, and the Canadian Naturopathic Association. Several members of the NIMH also practise in Canada an the USA.

Consultation and practice is much as in the UK, although there is widespread interest in both Native American remedies – such as golden seal and echinacea – and in the more exotic eastern remedies which frequently take on cult status especially in the over-the-counter market. Booming sales of kava (Piper methysticum) and the kombucha mushroom (Fungus japonicus), which is made into a mood-enhancing tea, have done little to endear establishment authorities to the credibility of herbal remedies.

The Health Protection branch of Health Canada has recently reclassified a number of traditional herbal remedies as drugs because of their proven pharmaceutical effects and may introduce fees for inspecting herbalists' stocks of "medicines" – a possibility which is causing practitioners in the area considerable concern. Several Canadian groups are currently campaigning for better regulation of herbal products.

Consulting a professional herbalist is not all that different from visiting a GP – or rather, visiting a GP as one would have done 40 or 50 years ago. Indeed, many herbalists liken their approach to that of the old-fashioned family physician, using a lot of patient listening and probing questions to uncover all the relevant symptoms, along with time-honoured diagnostic techniques: feeling pulses, looking at tongues, testing urine, and with clinical examinations dependent on palpation, auscultation and percussion rather than laboratory tests. A first consultation will generally take at least an hour and subsequent ones 20 minutes or so. A wide range of ailments is commonly treated: both the sort of problems one might normally take to a GP – infections, aches and pains, menstrual disorders, high

blood pressure, urinary dysfunction, digestive problems etc – and those chronic conditions for which herbalism is often seen as a "last resort", such as rheumatoid arthritis, ME, emphysema and so on.

As well as reviewing the current illness, the herbalist will ask about medical history – previous health problems that may be contributing to the current imbalance, family tendencies and allergies, diet, lifestyle, stresses and worries.

Examinations may include taking blood pressure and pulses, palpating the abdomen to identify the cause of pain or discomfort, listening to chest wheezes (auscultation) or checking the degree of movement in an arthritic knee or shoulder. Simple clinical tests undertaken on site could include urine analysis or measuring haemoglobin levels using a tiny drop of blood. Existing orthodox medication also needs to be checked.

Herbalists would certainly not recommend dropping vital drugs, but any incompatibility of these with herbal remedies obviously needs to be considered when prescribing plant medicines. Similarly, many patients turn to herbs because they are anxious to phase out their drugs, for whatever reason, and a safe programme of replacing them with gentler herbal remedies needs to be devised – preferably with the support and co-operation of the patient's GP. Herbal remedies, for example, can be very helpful for sufferers trying to break an addiction to tranquillisers or sleeping pills – or as alternatives for those suffering the side effects from non-steroidal anti-inflammatory drugs used for arthritis.

At the end of the consultation, the patient does not simply leave with a prescription for the local pharmacist to dispense. In Britain, few pharmacies are willing to stock the hundreds of tinctures, creams, oils, powders, capsules or dried herbs that the medical herbalist needs to keep in stock, so all medical herbalists are permitted under the 1968 Medicines Act and the Medicines (Retail Sale and Supply of Herbal Remedies) Order 1977, to make and dispense their own remedies. As well as a combination of herbs, specially selected to help the unique health problems of each individual, the patient may leave the consultation room with a list of dietary suggestions, foods to avoid or details of those to eat more of. There may be recommended relaxation routines to follow or Bach Flower Remedies to help emotional factors affecting physical well-being. Or perhaps the patient will be sent away with a small growing plant to bring a little love and beauty into their life. Whatever the remedy, healing is a two-way process and the patient must take responsibility for their own health

and actively participate in any cure. Those who expect a "magic pill" to solve their problems with little effort of their own, may be happier with orthodox therapies.

Generally herbalists like to see patients fairly soon after the first consultation to check on progress – perhaps after two or three weeks – with regular meetings every four to six weeks for six months or more in chronic cases. Herbal medication is likely to be altered slightly after each consultation to reflect changes in the condition.

Just as all patients are different, so too are all herbalists. Finding a practitioner with whom you feel empathy and whom you can trust can be just as important in treatment as taking the right herbs. Some herbalists follow a

semi-orthodox path, prescribing remedies to ease symptoms just as modern drugs do, others will focus on holistic treatments urging major lifestyle changes. Some will use only Western herbs, others a combination of Chinese or Ayurvedic remedies. Some will talk mainly of pathological conditions, others will suggest *Qi* stagnation, allergies or define just about anything in terms of emotional stress. Some will depend on the consulting couch and the results of clinical tests for diagnosis – others will swing a pendulum or try kinesiology. If possible, choose your practitioner by personal recommendation from like-minded friends to ensure a good relationship with someone who understands your problem and whom you can also understand.

further reading

Bartram, T. (1995) *Encyclopaedia of Herbal Medicine*, Grace Publishers, Christchurch
Bown, D. (1995) *Encyclopaedia of Herbs and their Uses*, Dorling Kindersley, London
Brooke, E. (1992) *A Woman's Book of Herbs*, The Women's Press, London
Castelvetro, G. (translated by G. Riley, 1989) *The Fruits, Herbs and Vegetables of Italy*, Viking, London
Chancellor, P. M. (1971) *Handbook of the Bach Flower Remedies*, C. W. Daniels, Saffron Walden
Chevallier, A. (1993) *Herbal First Aid*, Amberwood Publishing, Christchurch
Chevallier, A. (1996) *Encyclopaedia of Medicinal Plants*, Dorling Kindersley, London
Davis, P. (1995) *Aromatherapy: An A-Z, 2nd Edition*, C. W. Daniels, Saffron Walden.
Erasmus, U. (1986) *Fats and Oils*, Alive Books, Canada
Foster, S., and Yue, C. (1992) *Herbal Emissaries*, Healing Arts Press, Rochester, Vermont
Frawley, D., and Lad, V. (1986) *The Yoga of Herbs*, Lotus Press, Santa Fe

Frawley, D. (1989) *Ayurvedic Healing: A Comprehensive Guide*, Passage Press, Salt Lake City, Utah
Grieve, M. (1931) *A Modern Herbal*, Jonathan Cape, London
Griggs, B. (1981) *Green Pharmacy*, Jill Norman & Hobhouse, London
Gursche, S. (1993) *Healing with Herbal Juices*, Alive Books, Canada
Harrison, J. (1984) *Love Your Disease*, Angus & Robertson, Sydney
Hobbs, C. (1995) *Medicinal Mushrooms*, Botanica Press, Santa Cruz
King, F. X. (1986) *Rudolf Steiner and Holistic Medicine*, Rider, London
Leung, A. Y. (1985) *Chinese Herbal Remedies*, Wildwood House, London
Maury, M. (1974) "How to cure yourself with wine" in Montignac, M. (1991) *Dine Out and Lose Weight*, Editions Artulan, Paris
McIntyre, A. (1988) *Herbs for Pregnancy and Childbirth*, Sheldon Press, London
Mills, S. Y. (1991) *Out of the Earth*, Viking, London
Newell C. A., Anderson, L. A., and

Phillipson, J. D. (1996) *Herbal Medicines*, The Pharmaceutical Press, London
Ody, P. (1993) *The Herb Society's Complete Medicinal Herbal*, Dorling Kindersley, London
Ody, P. (1995) *The Herb Society's Home Herbal*, Dorling Kindersley, London
Ody, P. (1996) *Handbook of Over-the-Counter Herbal Medicines*, Kyle Cathie, London
Tang, S, and Craze, R (1995) *Chinese Herbal Medicine*, Piatkus, London
Tisserand, R. (1977) *The Art of Aromatherapy*, C. W. Daniels, Saffron Walden
Vogel, V. J. (1970) *American Indian Medicine*, University of Oklahoma Press
Weiss, R. F. (1988) *Herbal Medicine*, Beaconsfield Publishers, Beaconsfield
Wren, R. C. (1988) *Potter's New Cyclopaedia of Botanical Drugs and Preparations*, C. W. Daniels, Saffron Walden

useful addresses

UK
Associations and professional bodies

British Herbal Medicine Association, Sun House, Church Street, Stroud, Gloucestershire GL5 1JL

The General Council and Register of Consultant Herbalists, Marlborough House, Swanpool, Falmouth, Cornwall TR11 4HW

The Herb Society, 134 Buckingham Palace Road, London SW1W 9SA

National Institute of Medical Herbalists, 56 Longbrook Street, Exeter, Devon EX4 6AH

The Natural Medicines Group, PO Box 5, Ilkeston, Derbyshire DE7 8LX

The Register of Chinese Herbal Medicine, PO Box 400, Wembley, Middlesex HA9 9NZ

School of Phytotherapy, Bucksteep Manor, Bodle Street Green, Hailsham, East Sussex

Mail order herb suppliers

G Baldwin & Co, 171-174 Walworth Road, London SE17 1RW

Dorwest Herbs, Shipton Gorge, Bridport, Dorset DT6 4LP

East West Herbs Ltd, Langston Priory Mews, Kingham, Oxon OX7 6UW

Galen Herbal Supplies Ltd, Unit 17, St David's Industrial Estate, Pengam, Blackwood, Gwent NP2 1SW

Hambledon Herbs, Court Farm, Milverton, Somerset TA4 1NF

Hartwood Aromatics, Enterprise House, Courtauld's Way, Coventry, West Midlands CV6 5NX

Herbs of Grace, 5 Turnpike Road, Red Lodge, Bury St Edmunds, Suffolk IP28 8JZ

Neal's Yard Remedies, 5 Golden Cross, Cornmarket Street, Oxford OX1 3EU.

Nurseries and specialist suppliers

Barwinnock Herbs, Barrhill, Ayrshire KA26 0RB

Brin School Fields, The Old School, Flichity, Inverness

Cheshire Herbs, Fourfields, Forest Road, Little Budworth, Tarporley, Cheshire CW6 9ES

Hollington Nurseries, Woolton Hill, Newbury, Berks RG20 9XT

Iden Croft Herbs, Frittenden Road, Staplehurst, Kent TN12 0DN

The Cottage Herbery, Mill House, Boraston, Tenbury Wells, Worcs WR15 8LZ

The Herb Farm, Peppard Road, Sonning Common, Reading RG4 9NJ

The Herb Garden, Hall View Cottage, Hardstoft, Pilsley, Chesterfield, Derbyshire

Australia
Associations and schools

National Herbalists' Association of Australia, Suite 14, 247-249 Kingsgrove Road, Kingsgrove, NSW 2208

School of Herbal Medicine/Phytotherapy, PO Box 5310, Toowoomba, Queensland 4350

Southern Cross Herbal School, PO Box 734, Gosford, NSW 2250

Southern School of Natural Therapies, 43 Victoria Street, Fitzroy, Victoria 3065

Victorian Herbalists' Association, 24 Russell Street, Northcote, Victoria 3070

Mail order herb suppliers

Australian Botanical Products Pty Ltd, 39 Melverton Drive, Hallam, Victoria 3803

Blackmores Ltd, 23 Roseberry Street, Balgowlah, NSW 2093

Greenridge Botanicals, PO Box 1197, Toowoomba, Queensland 4350

Essential Therapeutics, 6 Stuart Road, Lilydale, Victoria 3140

Herbs of Gold Pty Ltd, 120 Milwood Avenue, Chatswood, NSW 2067

Medi-Herb Pty Ltd, PO Box 713, Warwick, Queensland 4370

Southern Light Herbs, PO Box 227, Maldon, Victoria 3463

in**dex**

photographic **acknowledgements**

The author and publishers would like to thank Laura Hodgson for her contribution to this book, and the individuals and agencies listed below for permission to reproduce copyright photographs.

Key:
LH: Laura Hodgson
GPL: Garden Picture Library
Holt: Holt Studios International
HA: Heather Angel
JF: John Fielding
JM: Jekka McVicar

p .1 GPL/John Glover
p. 2 LH
p. 15 GPL/Marianne Majerus
p. 20 LH
p. 23 LH
p. 27 LH
p. 28 LH
p. 31 LH
p. 33 LH
p. 35 LH
p. 37 LH
p. 39 LH
p. 41 LH

p.. 44 Holt/Nigel Cattlin
p. 51 GPL/John Glover
p. 53 GPL/David Askham
p. 55 GPL/Jerry Pavia
p. 60 HA
p. 62 GPL/Laslo Puskas
p. 63 GPL/Howard Rice
p. 65 GPL/John Glover
p. 66 HA
p. 70 GPL/Geoff Dann
p. 73 Holt/Nigel Cattlin
p. 77 JF
p. 79 JF
p. 83 JM
p. 85 HA
p. 87 Holt/Nigel Cattlin
p. 89 Holt/Inga Spence
p. 91 top left: Holt/Nigel Cattlin; top right: HA; bottom left: GPL/Michel Viard; Bottom right: Holt/Nigel Cattlin
p. 94 Holt/Nigel Cattlin
p. 96 GPL/Mayer/Le Scanff
p. 99 GPL/Bob Challinor
p. 107 top left GPL/John Glover; top right Holt/Bob Gibbons; bottom left GPL/Neil Holmes; bottom right GPL/Mayer/Le Scanff
p. 113 HA

p. 116 Holt/Nigel Cattlin
p. 117 Holt/Bob Gibbons
p. 119 top left Holt/Nigel Cattlin; top right HA; bottom left: Holt/Bob Gibbons; bottom right GPL/Philippe Bonduel
p. 122 top left Holt/Nigel Cattlin; bottom left GPL/John Glover; bottom right Holt/Nigel Cattlin
p. 125 top left GPL/J. S. Sira; top right Holt/Bob Gibbons; bottom left: GPL/Geoff Dann; bottom right Holt/Nigel Cattlin
p. 129 top left GPL/Brian Carter; top right Holt/Jean Hall; bottom left Holt/Nigel Cattlin; bottom right HA
p. 131 Holt/Bob Gibbons
p. 133 top left GPL/David Russell; top right GPL/Geoff Dann; bottom left Holt/Bob Gibbons; bottom right Holt/Duncan Smith
p. 134 Holt/Nigel Cattlin
p. 137 top left Holt/Jean Hall; top right GPL/Roger Hyam; bottom left HA; bottom right Holt/Nigel Cattlin
p. 139 top GPL/J. S. Sira; bottom Holt/Nigel Cattlin
p. 141 Holt/Nigel Cattlin
p. 143 LH
p. 145 top left Holt/Duncan Smith; top right HA; bottom left Holt/Nigel Cattlin; bottom right Holt/Nigel Cattlin

040-873-1